VEGAN NUTRITION:
PURE and SIMPLE

by MICHAEL KLAPER, M.D.

**Printed
on
Recycled Paper**

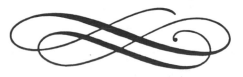

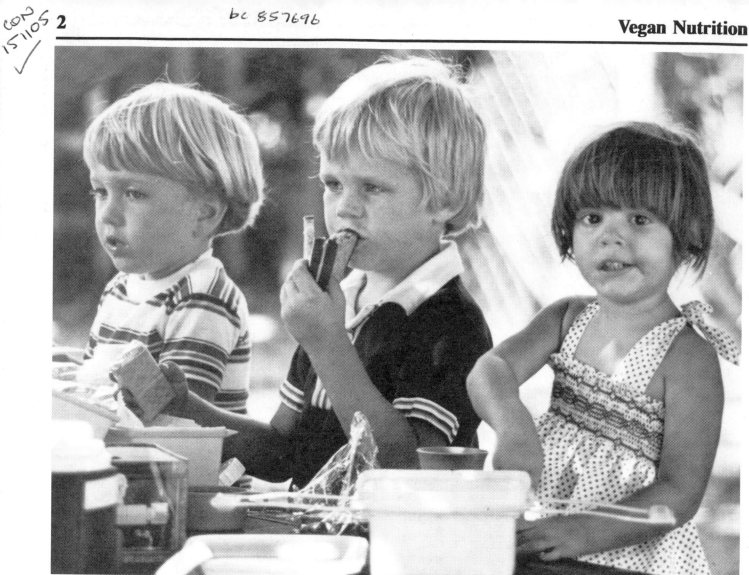

JUDY SUMMERS

NOTICE TO READERS

The information in this book is intended to serve as a guideline to help plan an adequate nutritional program free of meat, dairy, and other animal products, for adults in good health. The nutritional values cited are accepted averages derived for the general population from accredited nutritional sources. Should any physical condition exist requiring medical treatment of special consideration, nutritional advice from the appropriate professional (M.D., R.D., etc.) should be sought. Do not change medications without consulting the proper health professional.

Fourth Edition
©Copyright 1997, 1994, 1992, 1987
ISBN 0-9614248-9-3
GENTLE WORLD, INC.
P.O. Box 110
Paia, Maui, HI 96779

FOREWORD FOR HEALTH PROFESSIONALS

Among those physicians, dietitians, and others with a professional interest in nutrition and health, there may be some who are not familiar with pure vegetarian (vegan) nutrition. Some may question the suitability of such a dietary approach, especially for pregnant women and growing children. **VEGAN NUTRITION: PURE and SIMPLE** presents the rationale for animal-free nutrition, and a guide to its proper application in healthy adults. The author's **PREGNANCY, CHILDREN, AND THE VEGAN DIET** describes vegan nutrition for pregnant women and children.

The increasing importance of the role of vegetarian nutrition in modern life makes this book of special value to the health practitioner and nutrition counselor.

We now live in a world of Salmonella-tainted chickens, Listeria-covered cheese, and beefburgers laced with estrogenic hormones and residues of potent antibiotics. These are **very good reasons** why people would want to obtain their daily nourishment without pouring fatty and contaminated meat and dairy products through their bloodstream every few hours.

Many people are concerned about the high incidence of health threats that are linked to improper diet, like heart attacks, strokes, birth defects, breast, prostate and other cancers, high blood pressure, diabetes and other diseases. They are seeking more wholesome food alternatives for themselves and their families.

Some concerned people do not want to contribute to the violence inherent in meat production, such as that inflicted upon animals during factory farming, or at the slaughterhouse. Still others hope to heal our planet's troubled ecosystem, with its vanishing rain forests and dwindling water supplies, by utilizing the vegan nutritional approach. Thus, for many reasons, the awareness of the advantages of a flesh-free diet is rapidly increasing, as are the numbers of those who are benefiting from its practice.

The practice of pure vegetarian nutrition is an established and growing reality. People around the planet are thriving on a vegan-style diet, having healthy babies and raising children, as they have done throughout history.[1] As vegetarians are encountered in clinical practice, a knowledge of the principles of animal-free nutrition is helpful to professionals in understanding their clients' nutritional strategies, and in planning health-promoting diet choices.

The rationale for pure vegetarian nutrition is supported by sound scientific principles. The clinician and nutritionist should feel comfortable with the fact that it is physiologically and biochemically possible (and even easy) for people to properly nourish themselves on a diet **free** of animal products.

The body of Homo sapiens has no nutritional requirement for the flesh of animals, for the eggs of chickens, or for the milk of cows. A brief review of biochemical principles will confirm that humans can derive all of their essential nutrients from a plant-based diet.

Human health and growth requires sufficient supplies of the following essential nutrients:

1. **Carbohydrates** } Energy
2. **Fats** } (calories)
3. **Protein**
4. **Vitamins**
5. **Minerals**
6. **Water**

Considering each nutrient individually, most of the body's **energy** needs are met by 2-carbon acetate groups that feed the Krebs citric acid cycle. The energy is stored as adenosine triphosphate (ATP). The (2-carbon) "cell fuel" for this process abounds in the **carbohydrates** and **fats** found in the starches, sugars, and oils in grains, potatoes, fruits, nuts, and seeds. A well-planned vegan diet amply supplies adequate calories.

The two essential **fatty acids**, linoleic acid and linolenic acid, needed for normal **fat** metabolism, are found abundantly in nuts, seeds, grains, and cooking oils.

All the essential amino acids required for human **protein** metabolism are contained in the high-quality proteins in grains, legumes, seeds, nuts, and green vegetables - and without undue concern for "protein combining."

All essential **vitamins** and **minerals** are found in green and yellow vegetables, and in fruits. In individual cases, selected vitamin and mineral supplementation (B-12, calcium, etc.) may be deemed necessary; these can be conveniently supplied through non- animal sources. (See "VITAMINS").

Thus, three balanced vegan meals daily, based upon grains, legumes, vegetables, fruits, nuts and seeds, will provide ample amounts of all the above nutrients for adults (pregnant or not) and growing children.

More and more people are seeking information on a plant- based diet, as it offers the promise of better health, and a safer, more plentiful world for themselves and their children. (See "The Future...In Our Hands").

VEGAN NUTRITION: PURE and SIMPLE is offered to professionals and the public to help in this important and timely educational process.

Michael Klaper, M.D.

Dedicated to Gentleness

...and the dream of a world in balance,
where human and non-human animals have nothing to fear.

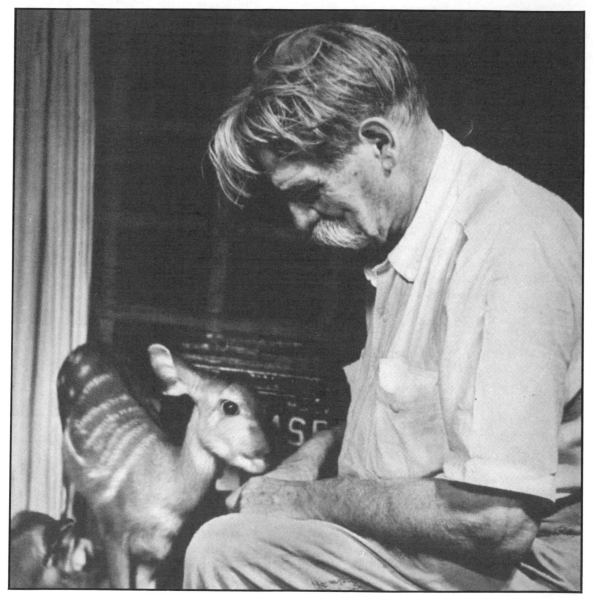

ERICA ANDERSON

DR. ALBERT SCHWEITZER
Physician/Humanitarian

*"No single phase of my own philosophy is more
representative of my thinking than 'Reverence for Life.'"*

*"I am conscious that flesh eating is NOT in accordance
with the finer feelings, and I abstain from it . . . "*

TABLE OF CONTENTS

INTRODUCTION

VEGAN NUTRITION: PURE AND SIMPLE will be helpful to those just becoming familiar with vegetarian food choices, as well as to "seasoned" vegetarians who seek a scientific and practical validation of their non-violent food preferences.

Once one has learned to make a few different vegan dishes for breakfast, lunch, and dinner, emphasizing nutritional food combinations that maximize protein and vitamin intake, it becomes easy to make it through the eating day, enjoying delicious, balanced vegan meals.

The evolving of each person's diet away from animal flesh is an effective strategy for improving individual health, as well as for solving our world's grave ecological problems. **VEGAN NUTRITION: PURE AND SIMPLE** is offered as a a hopeful vision and a practical aid in helping to create a healthy world for us all.

PART ONE

NEW VIEWINGS

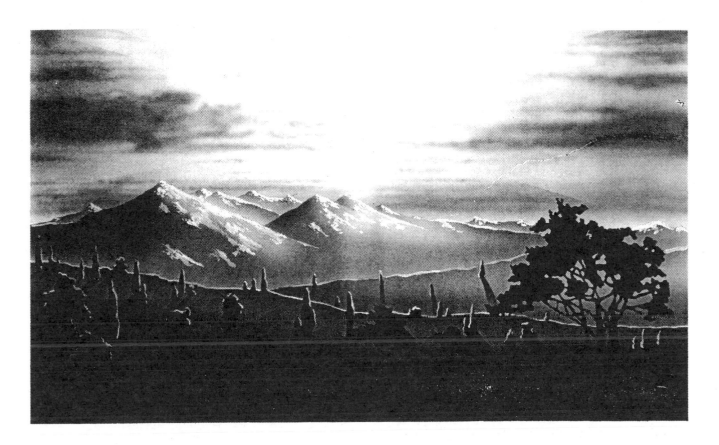

CHAPTER 1

PERSPECTIVES

In this time when food is processed, preserved, and irradiated, and so much is said about diet and nutrition, it is easy to become confused.

What does your body really need to function each day?

Are there any easy-to-follow rules and food patterns that will help you stay balanced and healthy, instead of increasing your susceptibility to disease?

Of course there are. The keys to balanced nutrition are easy to understand, and serve as powerful allies when put into practice.

Every day, we make many choices regarding what and when to eat. Although each individual food selec-tion may seem like a small one, the effect of our dietary choices over a lifetime is monumental. Second only to genetic inheritance, your daily food decisions are the greatest single determinant as to whether the body in which you live is lean, light, and healthy - moving free-ly without pain - or obese and sluggish, with high blood pressure, diabetes, narrow blood vessels, and a predisposition to cancers.

Each time we open our mouths to eat, we are making a decision and a statement. The silent ques-tions that we should consider, but often do not, are:

"Should I really eat this, or should I choose some-thing else?"

"Is the taste sensation I am about to have worth what this food, **and all it contains** is going to do to my body?"

If you are a pregnant woman or parent of young children, you might ask, "If I really love my child, do I want this food (or what is being called "food") to become part of his or her brain, heart, and body?"

How do you tell healthful foods from harmful ones?

Let's consider a few of the prevailing ideas about which foods are essential for good nutrition. We may find that some currently-held concepts are in need of revision...

The Rise and Fault of "THE BASIC FOUR"

For many of us, our nutrition education began and ended with a poster on the grammar school wall. The gist of the message delivered there was:

"Food comes in Four Food Groups"(and Four Food Groups only!) They are:

1) Meats,
2) Dairy,
3) Fruits & Vegetables, and
4) Grains.

Most of us were also taught that we require a portion from **each** group **every** day or we risk becoming ill, malnourished, or dead.

This "Basic Four Food Group" approach is still taught to American school children. It is the foundation of most diet planning in hospitals, in the military, in prisons, in government institutions, and in households across the country. Unfortunately, the "Basic Four" food scheme has little to do with the creation of good health in human beings.

How could it be a reliable guide to health? The "Basic Four" plan was not established upon firm, scientifically-based principles of human nutrition, but rather, upon the economics and politics of meat and dairy production.[2]

Let's explode a myth. The "Basic Four" scheme was **not** delivered to Moses on Mount Sinai, carved in stone along with the Ten Commandments. It was created by the United States Department of Agriculture (U.S.D.A.) in 1956. This was a most significant event in the history of Western nutrition, and we all still feel the consequences of that maneuver.

In 1930, there were twelve food groups (the "Basic Twelve"), but because that number proved to be too unwieldy for the public to use, they were narrowed to the "Basic Seven" in 1944.

From the early 1900's, heavy machinery and "favorable-interest" financing became accessible to American farmers. As they plowed freshly irrigated fields on new tractors fueled by inexpensive gasoline, huge amounts of grain and soybeans were produced, and fed to hundreds of millions of destined-to-be-eaten cows, pigs, chickens, and other animals.

Production of "destined-to-be-eaten" animals increased, and it became economically profitable to encourage Americans to eat more and more high-fat, high-protein, meat and dairy products. There then followed a great increase in the national consumption of animal flesh - and thus animal fat. Soon steep increases in the rates of heart disease, strokes and of other blood vessel diseases were observed.

By 1956, there were medical and nutritional studies appearing in the scientific literature, indicating that meat and dairy products were associated with severe degenerative diseases, like heart disease and strokes.[3] It had also been observed that people whose diets were based upon starches, fruits, and vegetables, lived longer, healthier lives.[4]

However, the overriding goal of the U.S.D.A. was (and is) to encourage the production of, and provide a strong and growing market for, agricultural products. So, despite medical reports to the contrary, and under the approving eyes of the meat and dairy industries, the "Basic Seven" was pared down to the "Basic Four". Suddenly, **one half** the food group choices presented to Americans by their government as "nutritious" were the body parts or nursing secretions of animals.

This is no small matter. Animal flesh is fundamentally different than plant tissue, in hundreds of subtle but crucial ways that affect human health:

1) The amounts and chemical kinds of **fats** in animals (cholesterol and triglycerides) are very different than those found in plants. Of great importance is the fact that only animal foods contain cholesterol. **No** plant contains cholesterol in any significant amount. The amount of cholesterol that pure vegetarians (vegans) eat in their diet each day is **zero**.[5]

This is perfectly fine, because your human body will make all the cholesterol it needs from essential fats found in whole grains, sunflower seeds, and other oil-rich foods. People following a vegan style of eating are usually lean, with cholesterol levels averaging well below 180 mg. percent. [6]

Meat fat is thicker, more "saturated," solid at body temperature, and far more likely to clog human arteries than plant oils. A balanced vegan diet usually creates normal blood cholesterol levels in all but those people with severe genetic disorders.[7]

2) The **protein** of animal muscle (steak, chicken meat, fish fillets, etc.) is far more **concentrated** than

the plant protein found in whole grains, legumes, and green vegetables. As will be described in the chapters that follow, this concentrated protein load can leach calcium from the bones, contributing to osteoporosis[8], and clog the kidney filters, leading to kidney failure[9].

3) Flesh foods and dairy products are completely lacking in plant **fiber**, essential for proper digestion by the human intestine.

4) The balance of the key metallic elements, **sodium** and **potassium**, is reversed between plant foods and animal flesh. That is, animal foods have far more sodium than potassium, while most all plants are normally potassium-rich and low in sodium. Because the sodium/potassium content of foods is probably a key determinant of high blood pressure, this may explain why this disease is rampant in the meat-eating ("high-sodium") population, and extremely rare among pure ("high-potassium") vegetarians.[10]

5) Other biological, physical, and chemical properties of flesh foods, like **electrical charge** and stimulation of **inflammatory substances** (prostaglandin 2E), induce noticeable signs of **metabolic stress** in the body.

After a meal of animal flesh:

a. The white blood count increases,[11]

b. The red blood cells become more "sticky" and "sludge" in small blood vessels,[12] and

c. Levels of anti-inflammatory hormones (cortisol) and sex hormones (estrogen, prolactin) increase.[13]

These indicators that animal foods may not be appropriate for human "fuel" have largely been ignored.

On a national level, the signs that a high fat, meat-based diet is unhealthy are blatant. Every minute, two Americans suffer heart attacks from fat-clogged arteries, and one of them dies. Clogged arteries to hearts and brains kill more Americans than any other disease. Considering the nature of animal fat, and the effect that pouring it through the human bloodstream day after day for years must have, it does not seem surprising that the arteries of most Americans show signs of clogging with atherosclerosis.

Animal fats are not the optimal energy source for most of our body cells to burn. Actually, they are an inferior "fuel" for our body's "engine," generating many acidic waste products when metabolized. Most of our body cells prefer to burn a fuel of carbohydrates, such as the sugars and starches found in fruits, vegetables, grains, and potatoes.

Consider this analogy:

If you put diesel fuel (kerosene) into a car that runs on gasoline, the oily diesel fuel will not burn cleanly. Kerosene will eventually clog the V-8 engine with a greasy sludge. Animal fats are to the human body as diesel fuel is to the V-8 engine. Tides of animal fat flowing through our "piping system" (arteries) will eventually clog the pipes - leading to heart attacks, strokes, and other disasters.

No artery-clogging plaque of atherosclerosis has ever been found to be composed of rice and vegetables. On the contrary, the pathologist's chemical analysis of the fatty plugs that are removed from arteries inevitably includes the terms, "saturated fat" and "cholesterol," which are predictable and hazardous components of a meat and dairy-based diet.[14]

Just how fatty is the current American-style diet? Following the classic "Basic Four" Food Groups plan, a full and "nutritious" day of eating could include:

A breakfast of bacon and eggs, and a glass of milk;

A lunch of a cheeseburger, french fries, and a milkshake, and

A dinner featuring beefsteak (or fried chicken or fish), with baked potatoes and sour cream.

Ice cream is often eaten for dessert, as well as chocolate candy or potato chips for snacks and treats.

Consider all the animal fat that lies in ambush within these meals. The egg yolks, bacon, and cheese, are heavy with triglycerides and cholesterol. Even more fats lurk in the flesh of the beefburger and dinner steak (or chicken breast or fish fillet), as well as in the butterfat in the sour cream, milkshake, and chocolate.

These foods contain a total of 287 grams of fat - that is, 65 teaspoons! - exceeding the R.D.A. by 441%. These meals also pack 1127 milligrams of cholesterol, smothering the R.D.A. of 250 milligrams by 451% ![15]

This eating style creates a flood of animal fat coursing through the bloodstream every three to four hours. After eating a cheeseburger and milkshake (or other fatty meal), the blood actually becomes greasy with animal fat - and stays that way for up to four hours.

If you were to stand outside of a fast food restaurant with a blood-drawing syringe and take blood samples of the patrons leaving after a typical meal, you would witness something remarkable.

When drawn into a glass tube, and allowed to stand and coagulate, blood separates into (1) a dark red clot on the bottom of the tube, and (2) a clear liquid layer, called "serum," that floats to the top. Normal serum is transparent yellow; you can see clear through it.

CLEAR SERUM   LIPEMIC SERUM

(OPAQUE WITH FAT)

AFTER A MEAL OF RICE AND VEGETABLES.

AFTER A MEAL OF CHEESEBURGER AND MILKSHAKE.

The person who has just eaten a fatty meal - like a cheeseburger and fries, a pizza, or scrambled eggs - would be shocked to see a sample tube of their own blood. Instead of the clear, clean, yellow serum floating above the dark red clot, they would see a thick white cap of greasy fats, bobbing opaquely above the serum, and adhering to the sides of the tube.

This phenomenon is called **lipemia,** and is a familiar and predictable sight to the bloodbank technologist working on the after-lunch shift. The technologist can easily tell who ate a high-fat lunch, merely by looking at the settled samples of blood in the test tubes. Though everyone's blood may not show quite so milky an appearance, everyone suffers a surge of fat through their bloodstream after every animal-based meal. Not even mountain lions eat animal fat every four hours like modern North American humans do.

Whether derived from the thigh muscle of a bull (steak), the flight muscles from a chicken's breast (white meat), or the stomach of a pig (bacon), animal muscle is animal muscle, and its heavy fats, concentrated protein, and lack of fiber, spell trouble for the human digestive system. Similarly, products made from cows' milk and chickens' eggs are fiberless masses of saturated fat and foreign animal protein. The anatomy of the human body is marvelously adapted to digest plant foods, but it tends to become clogged and diseased when given the flesh diet of the carnivores.

Over the past fifty years, the American diet has become top heavy with meat. At the turn of the century our grandparents ate a flesh meal far less often than we do today. Now, due to the mechanized pro-

duction of meat and dairy products, eating animal products three times a day or more is commonplace. Through the media, meat-eating is massively advertised through images that portray everything but an accurate picture of the true cost of each cheeseburger and ice cream cone.

Medical studies clearly show that the higher the consumption of meat and dairy products (the first two of the "Basic Four") in any nation, the more its people suffer from heart attacks, strokes, diabetes, and cancer of bowel, breast, and prostate gland.[16c] Conversely, nations whose dietary patterns are based upon fruits, vegetables and grains, inevitably have low incidences of all these diseases.

The effect of the 1956 United States Department of Agriculture's "Basic Four" declaration was profound. The nutritional recommendations were drastically imbalanced to favor animal flesh and dairy foods. Medical reports which warned of the hazards of meat, and favored greater consumption of fruits, vegetables, grains and legumes, were overshadowed by the promise of short-term gains for farmers and meat and dairy producers.

The price that the "Basic Four" plan of affluent eating has inflicted upon America has been staggering in human suffering, health care costs and lost productivity. If the nutrition planners in 1956 had a crystal ball, and could have gazed upon our present day eating habits, laden with fatty meats and no-fiber, high-sodium dairy products, and then if they could peer into modern hospitals to view the overflowing coronary care units, cancer wards, and surgical suites where diseased colons are removed and clogged arteries are bypassed, I feel they would have made another choice.

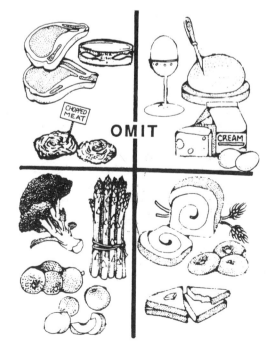

OMIT

CHAPTER 2

TAKING IT PERSONALLY
(and PROFESSIONALLY)

I have seen most of the faces of health and disease. After earning my medical degree in 1972 from the University of Illinois in Chicago, I took additional post-graduate training in surgery, anesthesia, obstetrics, and internal medicine. My clinical experience includes eight years of conventional general practice, and three years as physician in an isolated hospital in the mountains of northern California. I have practiced in emergency rooms and operating rooms as both surgeon and anesthetist, and have seen thousands of patients in my general medical office.

I see now that, like many of my colleagues, I undervalued the role of nutrition during my medical school education, and for much of my career in practice. I can empathize with those who feel the "Basic Four" plan is "proven and safe". We all grew up eating meat and drinking milk. Such an "All-American" diet kept the farmers producing and prosperous, it tasted good, and it seemed to work. . . or did it?

After years of witnessing patients suffering from arteries clogging with fat, hearts failing from high blood pressure, colons erupting with cancerous tumors and obesity-caused diabetes and arthritis, I looked again at the role of diet as a determinant of the diseases people brought to my office and operating table.

In medical school, I had delighted in learning about our amazingly efficient digestive system. Within minutes of eating **anything,** molecules of that substance flow through **every** cell in the body. How then, could I believe that what people eat plays no significant role in the creation of disease? Along with my clinical medical practice, I began to make a serious study of nutrition.

I re-examined the anatomy of our digestive system, and reviewed the biochemical and nutritional requirements of the human body (see PART TWO). I realized that HUMAN BEINGS HAVE NO NUTRITIONAL RE-QUIREMENTS FOR THE FLESH OR MILK OF ANIMALS.

Everything that humans require for growth and health comes from the delicious bounty that grows from the ground. The largest and most powerful animals on Earth, elephants, giraffes, bulls, and gorillas, grow to tremendous size, yet they **never** eat meat or drink the milk of a cow, let alone devour a cheese-and- pepperoni pizza!

As I came to understand the differences between animal flesh and plant foods, and thus comprehended more about the true nature of meat and diary products (see PART TWO) and what they do to the human body, I lost my desire to eat them.

Perhaps because much of my growing up was done on a dairy farm in Wisconsin, I was still drinking milk by the quart and eating cheese by the chunk. After seeing the fatty blood tubes from my meat and dairy-eating medical patients, I had a powerful realization:

Not only were my patients making their blood run thick with fat after a cheese sandwich or milkshake, but so, too, was I.

Suddenly, it became a case of "Physician, heal thyself." I went home and rid my refrigerator and pantry of meat, eggs, and dairy products. I found an excellent vegan cookbook and learned to make a few "sure-fire" breakfasts, lunches and dinners. The vast world of delicious vegan cuisine soon revealed itself, as well as the delights of shopping at the natural food store. It's been great eating ever since.

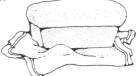

Within six weeks of eliminating animal products from my diet, I observed something wonderful happening within my body: namely, the 15 pound "spare tire" of fat around my waist had melted away, and my previous 138/88 blood pressure had settled to a comfortable 110/70. Living in a light, lean body had become a pleasure.

I had learned a powerful principle, and I soon began to use it to help my patients. I was able to counsel those who were overweight with a diet strategy that made sense:

"Stop running animal fat through your bloodstream, just for a few days or a week, and see how much better you feel."

"Derive your energy (calories) from the carbohydrates and oils in plants, rather than from the fat of animals."

"Base your diet on grains, legumes, fruits, and vegetables, take a brisk walk every day, (and smile a lot,) and you will become leaner and healthier!"

I soon realized that it is not enough to tell people what **not** to eat, but they must see (and taste!) foods free of animal flesh for themselves. Realizing that education is an essential part of healing, I arranged for a cook to come to my office and set up a small kitchen where we conducted meatless and dairyless cooking classes and demonstrations.

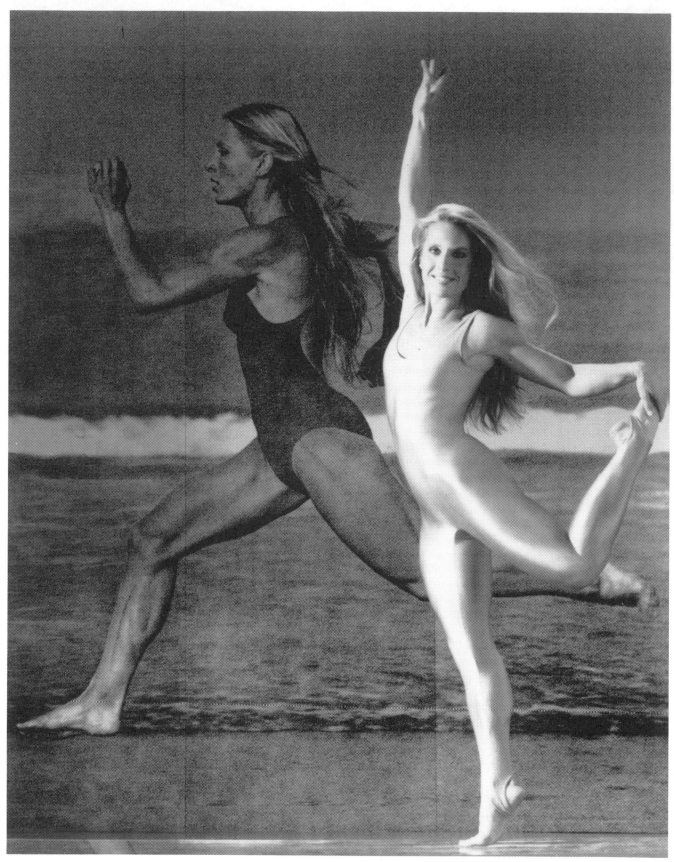

GAYLE OLINE KOVA
Marathon champion/Olympic Athlete

*" Vegetarianism is a deed of our hearts that will enable us to
leave behind a legacy of life and love for others."*

Soon I began to see welcome, but not unexpected, changes in my overweight patients. As they came in for their weekly weighings, those who followed the vegan diet, and enjoyed a twenty-minute walk every day, showed a steady downward progression of their weight, averaging two pounds per week.

Delightfully, they also experienced a similar downward progression of their high blood pressure measurements, cholesterol levels, and triglyceride counts. My diabetic patients achieved lower blood sugar levels, and I witnessed decreasing levels of uric acid in my patients with gout. Of course, I was then able to lower or discontinue many medications I had prescribed for these conditions. Some patients with high blood pressure, who had been told they would have to take blood pressure medication "for the rest of their life," became leaner, achieved normal blood pressures, and were able to stop their pills completely.

These benefits were predictable improvements in obesity-related disorders, like adult-onset diabetes and high blood pressure, observed as the patients' pounds of excess body fat melted away. Surprising to me, however, were the "unexpected" benefits that began to appear in many of these same patients. Chronic **inflammatory** conditions began to subside:

Arthritic people with red swollen joints noticed the redness and swelling diminish, and soon were able to move with less or no pain at all;

Eczema patients watched their skin clear;

Asthma patients with inflamed, swollen bronchial tubes found that they were able to breathe better, and that they required less medication. Some were able to discontinue their asthma medicine completely;

Female patients with premenstrual syndrome (PMS) found their symptoms greatly relieved when they eliminated animal protein and fat from their diet (thus lowering the level of cramp-inducing prostaglandins in their uterus muscle.)

Relief from these various inflammatory conditions appears to be a "bonus" that comes from the freeing of the human immune system from assaults by foreign animal proteins inherent in meat and dairy products. Apparently, fragments of animal protein find their way into the circulatory system after most every meal containing meat or dairy products. Antibodies against the protein in milk, as well as against beef muscle, are commonly found in the blood of omnivores.[16a] As the vegan diet eliminates the repeated immunologic insults from animal protein, (low-grade) inflammatory reactions in membranes throughout the body, including the joints, lungs, and skin, begin to subside.

I now expect (and usually see) rapid and sustained clinical improvement in most of my patients with obesity, high blood pressure, allergies, arthritis, and various inflammatory conditions, if they adopt and maintain a vegan style of nutrition. Within days of beginning to nourish their bodies with a pure plant-based fuel, most people feel lighter and "cleaner," and experience more energy and a heightened sense of well-being.

When necessary in my practice, I do prescribe medication and make recommendations for surgery. There are cases where dietary changes alone are not sufficient to correct the particular imbalance. However, following surgical or medical intervention, the patient must learn to make appropriate food choices in order to create and sustain true health.

I am convinced that a proper diet is essential for maintaining or regaining one's physical well-being. It would seem that the converse is also true: an unbalanced diet, top heavy with fat, protein, and toxins like cigarettes, drugs, and alcohol, stifles health and is the foundation of many of the diseases seen in Western countries today. The time has arrived when people must take these facts and observations seriously, and re-examine their own diets and lifestyles.

Every person is in charge of their own "Department of Nutrition," and, given the right guidelines, can make the best choices for themselves. One can benefit from the experience of the "Great American Dietary Catastrophe," and avoid the mistakes made by others. Even if you have been following a "junk food diet" for many years, it is never too late to begin to halt, or actually reverse, body damage that has been inflicted through unbalanced nutrition.

As hazards of meat and dairy products reveal themselves, many authorities advocate "moderating" their intake. However, when one considers reducing the body's burden of harmful substances, (like animal flesh and cow's milk products are showing themselves to be), "moderation" does not produce the highest level of health. There is strong medical evidence that complete freedom from eating animal flesh and cow's milk products, a vegan approach to nutrition, is a gateway to optimal nutritional health.[17]

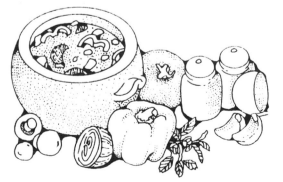

CHAPTER 3

A TASTE IS WORTH A THOUSAND WORDS

The reader may be aware that there is reluctance on the part of many reputable physicians and nutritionists to recommend vegan nutrition as a (the?) standard diet. In the past, scientific articles about vegan nutrition have often been accompanied by suggestions of, and warnings about, possible deficiencies in vital nutrients.[18] Old concepts can linger long, and despite years of successful clinical experience with vegan nutrition, and the mounting evidence that documents its efficacy, a few doubts remain in the minds of some nutrition planners and researchers.

These scientists can take comfort in the safety of vegan nutrition if they review some basic principles of biochemistry and human physiology. These sciences tell us that an easily- planned, balanced, plant-based diet, with vitamin supplementation if deemed necessary[19], is entirely adequate for full human nutrition, as presented in the "Foreword for Health Professionals," and in PART THREE.

The education of nutritional professionals is grounded in the doctrine of the "Basic Four Food Groups." This makes it difficult for Western-trained nutritionists to conceive of a healthy human diet free of the meat and milk of animals. This belief persists despite the fact that, as stated earlier, people have been thriving on animal-free diets for thousands of years, and do so today, often at higher levels of individual and national health than average North Americans.

Despite concerns of nutritionists, deficiencies of protein, calcium, and vitamins are extremely rare in North American vegetarians. Far more rampant are the **diseases of excess** that plague meat-eating Americans due to overconsumption of fat and protein.

Few of the authorities expressing reservations about vegan nutrition have ever had the experience of meeting a vegan person, or seeing a healthy, active, growing vegan child. They have not yet witnessed the health enhancing effects of a pure, plant-based diet upon the human body. (The likelihood of such a meeting increases daily, however, as more people discover the benefits of vegan nutrition - seven million people in North America now call themselves "vegetarian," and the numbers are growing rapidly.)

In addition, many who teach and write about nutrition have never tasted well-prepared vegan food. A welcome discovery awaits them as they learn how satisfying and nutritious a meal can be without a piece of animal muscle at its centerpiece.

For the scientist or clinician, the need for clinical validation is recognized. Clinical studies published in the medical literature show that a balanced vegan diet, with animal- free vitamin supplementation, or food fortification, when appropriate, is fully health supporting for adults and children.[20]

In their pioneering studies, Drs. Frey Ellis[21] and T.A.B. Sanders[22] also documented that vegan mothers have successful pregnancies, and raise healthy, bright, strong vegan children.[23] A recent medical study of 775 pregnant vegan women demonstrated that they had normal pregnancies, with a lower incidence of preeclampsia ("toxemia") and gave birth to healthy children.[23a] As previously mentioned, vegan nutrition greatly reduces the risk of many degenerative diseases that plague our society today.[24]

Another impressive validation of the advantages of vegan nutrition is being created by the strength and endurance of world-class vegetarian athletes who are setting new records in competitive sports, like triathalon champion "Ironman" Dave Scott, marathon swimmer, Marine Captain Alan Jones, marathon runner and fitness specialist, Gayle Olinekova, tennis professional, Peter Burwash, and Japanese baseball champions, the Seibu Lions.[25]

In the medical world, relief from serious diseases through the vegan eating style is no longer viewed as "miraculous". Reports of vegan nutrition used to control asthma[26], arthritis[27], angina[28], and other severe medical conditions, continue to appear in numerous medical journals.[29] As reported in "Lancet" in July, 1990, Dr. Dean Ornish has used an essentially vegan diet, along with exercise, stress reduction, and other techniques, to non-surgically help arteries reopen.

Even health organizations like the American Cancer Society and the American Heart Association recognize that the trend towards less animal products is a wise one for the nation. Their current advertising campaigns, encouraging low fat meals with (cancer-inhibiting) cruciferous and leafy green vegetables, reflect a new-found appreciation for a more vegetarian cuisine.

Nutrition is not a matter to be taken lightly. We must each seriously consider our responsibility for learning the fundamentals of what our bodies require, and what foods will meet these requirements. This is especially important for pregnant women, growing children, and those with disease or imbalances in the body.

The need to obtain your nutrients should **never** be a rationale for resorting to animal flesh or dairy products. Safer, nourishing plant sources are available that offer the key not only to health for individuals, but for planet Earth, as well...

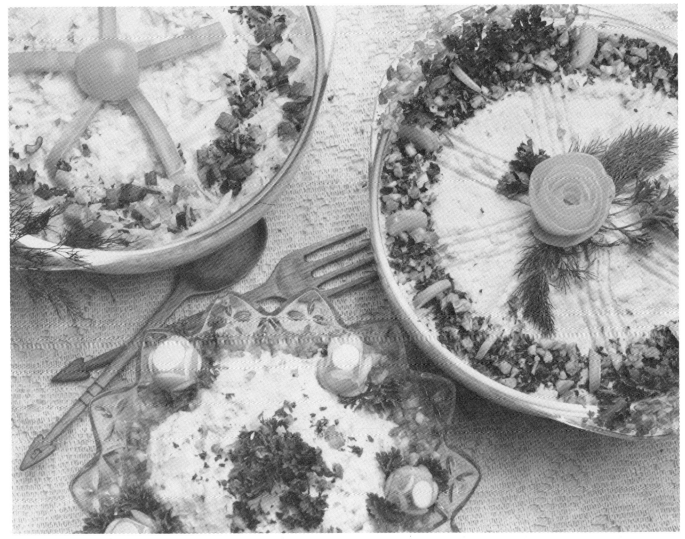

"My refusing to eat flesh occasioned an inconveniency, and I was frequently chided for my singularity, but, with this lighter repast, I made the greater progress, from greater clearness of head and quicker comprehension.
BEN FRANKLIN

CHAPTER 4

THE FUTURE . . . IN OUR HANDS

If everyone in America adopted a vegan style of eating, what would happen to the farmers and ranchers? What would happen to the cows? What would happen to the world?

The time has come to re-evaluate the role of meat and dairy production and consumption in the United States today.

More and more people in the meat and slaughter-related industries are becoming aware of the many problems associated with their products. The health problems stem from the fatty, fiberless nature of meat itself, as well as from the bacterial and chemical contamination inherent in modern factory farming methods. (See PART TWO.)

Yet, the scope of the problems resulting from the national craving for animal flesh and cow's milk,(two completely non- essential substances for human health), goes far beyond epidemics of Salmonella food poisoning. The economic, political and ecologic consequences of continuing the current rate of meat consumption are staggering, and threaten to create an ecologic catastrophe or to bring the world to the brink of nuclear war.

Consider the true cost of every hamburger eaten:

Growing animal tissue is terribly wasteful of **energy.** Cows, bulls and pigs are very inefficient converters of grain energy into edible flesh. Most of the food energy they take in is turned into edible body parts like bones and hair, or lost as heat while just walking around and breathing. Thus, it takes 16 pounds of high protein corn and soybeans to create one pound of feed lot beef flesh for a steak dinner.[30]

As a result of this energy inefficiency, current Western meat agriculture and food distribution devour billions of gallons of oil, in the form of diesel fuel and gasoline, to:

  run the tractors to grow the mountains of grain needed to feed the animals,

  fuel the trucks that ship the grains and animals,

  pump billions of gallons of water to irrigate fields and run the slaughter house operations, and

  power refrigeration units to keep the carcasses from decomposing.

Consider what a poor return meat yields in exchange for precious fuel oil invested: **60 calories** of petroleum energy must be **"plowed into the soil"** to **harvest one** food calorie from animal flesh. By contrast, growing grains and legumes to feed directly to people will **yield twenty** calories of food energy for each **one** calorie of fuel energy **invested.**[31] One acre of land will yield 165 pounds of beef, or 20,000 pounds of potatoes!

The current energy gluttony, driven by meat consumption, makes American agriculture, and thus the food supply of Americans, dependent upon a string of oil tankers stretching from our shores to the Persian Gulf - with all the political and military tensions that such dependency creates. Evolving to a plant-based diet would significantly reduce, or perhaps completely eliminate, our current addiction to imported oil. This could occur as huge tracts of land, freed from growing animal fodder, could be devoted to producing fast-growing trees or fiber plants to be harvested and burned for electricity and heat. As one pound of wood or other high-cellulose biomass contains 8500 BTU per pound, one acre of harvested biomass can replace approximately thirteen barrels of oil.

Burning biomass for energy is far more environmentally benign than burning fossil fuels. Trees and prairie grass are made from carbon dioxide taken from the air itself: burning this biomass only recycles atmospheric carbon dioxide and adds no net CO_2 to the air. Fossil fuels, like coal, oil, and gas, dredge up long-buried carbon deposits, out of the carbon cycle for millions of years, and, when burned, add fresh carbon dioxide to the atmosphere - retaining the Earth's heat, worsening problems with global warming and threatening to produce famine-causing weather abberations.

Thus, adoption of a more vegan style of nutrition on a national level could not only reduce our oil imports, but ease political and ecologic pressures as well.

WATER WORRIES

The extended and devastating droughts across North America in the summer of 1988, underscored one of the most wasteful and damaging aspects of the national meat habit: livestock production and slaughterhouse activity are, by far, the greatest **consumers,** and the most profligate **polluters** of **fresh water** in America today-soaking up **half** of all water consumed on the continent and polluting more water than all cities and industries combined.

Meat production requires gluttonous amounts of irrigation water to grow feedgrain, vast feedlots of large, thirsty animals that must be watered, and huge slaughterhouse operations awash in blood and entrails that flush through millions of gallons of drinking water per minute. Meanwhile, life-giving water tables across North America are falling steadily,[32] and wells across the country are going dry. [33]

Livestock meat production is also the most egregious polluter of fresh water in the world. In the United States, human beings create 12,000 pounds of excrement every second - while American livestock generate 250,000 pounds of excrement each second. A large livestock feeding operation, with 100,000 cows, has a sewage disposal problem of the same magnitude as the city of New Orleans. When the rain falls on the feedlots, tons of excrement can be washed into the nearest river, polluting untold billions of gallons of precious drinking water, often upstream from cities and towns.[34]

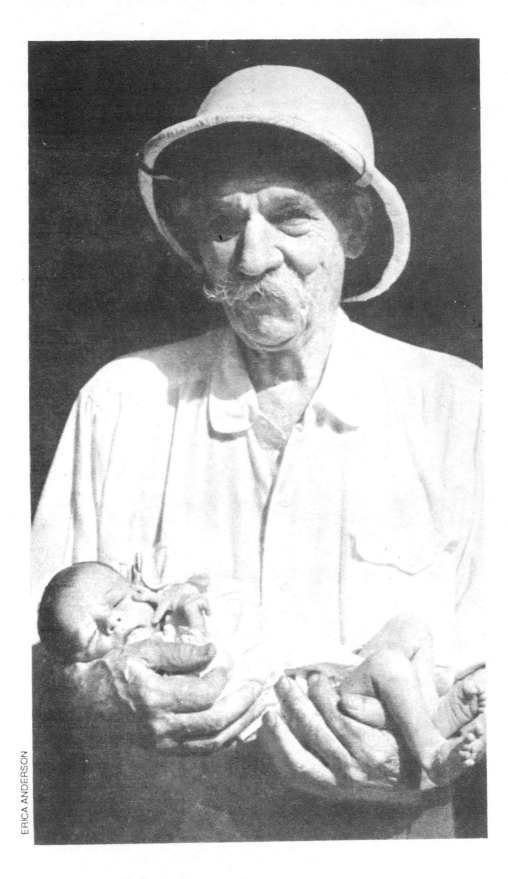

ERICA ANDERSON

ALBERT SCHWEITZER, M.D., PHD.
Doctor of Medicine; Doctor of Music; of Philosophy; of Theology

"Whenever I injure any kind of life, I must be quite certain that it is necessary. I must never go beyond the unavoidable, not even in apparently insignificant things. That man is truly ethical who shatters no ice crystal as it sparkles in the sun, tears no leaf from a tree ... "

This year twenty million people will starve to death due to lack of grains and legumes to eat. A child on our planet starves to death every three seconds.[36] If Americans decrease their meat consumption by only ten per cent, enough land would be freed to grow food for every person on Earth who would otherwise starve to death this year.[37] The solution to world hunger is to help other nations prosper, helping them to control their populations and grow their own food. However, in the short term, the exploding human populations and dwindling farmlands will force us to grow more grain for direct human consumption and less, if any, for the grain-feeding of animals.

The American "hamburger obsession" exacts another grave price, affecting all life forms on this planet. In order to harvest timber and grow "cash crop beef," to maximize profits and reduce foreign debt, vast tracts of priceless, tropical rainforests are being cut and burned at the staggering rate of twenty acres per minute, twenty-four hours a day. This equals a forest area the size of Pennsylvania disappearing every year. This relentless destruction of rain forests also obliterates three entire species of rare plants and animals every day, including the loss of plants with potentially great medicinal benefits.

Whether Americans actually import and consume "rainforest beef" or merely set the example for others through our prodigious beef consumption, our meat habit is a driving force of ecologic destruction.

Nothing fouls the streams like wallowing cows, and nothing turns grassland to desert wasteland like beef and dairy cattle grazing upon the hillsides. Stripped of the grasses and trees, the topsoil of land grazed on by cattle quickly erodes and washes into the rivers with every rainstorm. The United States taxpayer subsidizes cattle grazing on National Forest and other public lands. The cattle producer pays but a minimal grazing fee - a trivial portion of the cost of repairing the habitat destruction wrought by grazing thousands of heads of cattle upon the fragile, semi-arid ecosystems of the American West.

Almost half of America's croplands are devoted to producing feedcorn, soybeans, oats, sorghum, bay, and other animal fodder. Because the majority of the six billion tons of priceless topsoil that erodes off American farmlands yearly blows and washes off grazing lands or these vast fields of animal food, meat production, driven by our animal-based diet, is responsible for the vast majority of future-threatening topsoil erosion. This pernicious loss of topsoil is completely arrestable - the floor of a healthy forest does not erode. It is time to reconsider other uses for the fertile lands and soils of North America - while we still have them.[40]

As author John Robbins states in **DIET FOR A NEW AMERICA**, 'We do not inherit the land from our ancestors, we borrow it from our children." The American meat habit is squandering our children's priceless inheritance.[41] Of extreme importance, the growing spectre of world **starvation** makes the American meat habit especially grotesque. Eighty per cent of all the grains and legumes grown in America today becomes food, not for hungry human beings, but for animals![35] The grain and water resources that are converted into a single beefsteak meal can feed eight people for a day.

American forests are also continually disappearing under the chainsaw and bulldozer blade, turning much of our national wilderness heritage into cow pastures and cattle-watering holes.[39] We are trading our forests for cheeseburgers and hot dogs. Many people on Earth are now realizing that in the late twentieth century on Planet Earth the raising and killing of animals for food has become far too costly.

Fortunately, all the problems which seem to be dragging us along a collision course to disaster can be reversed and transformed into forces of rescue, beginning with a simple realization. It is time to positively change our taste preferences, and begin to make food choices in harmony with the nutritional realities of our bodies, and the ecological balance of nature.

It is no coincidence that **precisely** the same evolution to plant-based food choices that will improve the health of each person, will also help to rebalance the natural (and man-made) systems of planet Earth.

As less meat is produced and consumed, land will be freed for the great forests of our continent to return - and as they do, the water will become cleaner and more plentiful. As oil burning in animal agriculture decreases, the air will become clearer. Every person who changes to a pure vegetarian diet saves one acre of trees.[42]

Most of the erosion of our topsoil and much of the poisoning of our air, water, and other life-support systems would cease - and a deep healing of the Planet would begin.

Human suffering from degenerative diseases resulting from an animal-based diet should diminish, and soon following, the national financial burden of medical costs and high taxes will lessen.

With lower health care costs, lending money would become available to help people build new houses, schools, and non-polluting energy sources . The national debt would decrease, as should our taxes.

World hunger could and should disappear. Only economics and politics would (temporarily) prevent the available food from actually finding its way into the mouths of the hungry.

A new era of peace and plenty could dawn for all the Earth's inhabitants.[43]

...probably dependent upon, Homo sapiens, at this time in his history, evolving past the taste for animal flesh.

What of the people presently making their living from meat and dairy production? Farmers, ranchers, and meat producers are not "the enemy" in the "nutrition battle" or the "ecology war." Rather, they are valued friends and family members, people who need our help to become aware of the true cost and ecological effects of the products they create - and to help them transition to creating product free of hidden costs, to human health or to the Planet.

A reaffirmation of the farmer's role as "the good steward of the land" is in order. There many wonderful things one can do with vast open ranges and fields; we don't have to run cattle on the land. One can raise food crops for humans, like high-protein grains, legumes, and greens, as well as bountiful fruit orchards and nut groves, succulent vegetables, medicinal herbs, or jojoba beans, with their wonderful (and valuable) lubricating oil. Healthy forests yield lumber, fiber, paper, fuel, fresh water, vigorous wildlife, and oxygen. An acre of healthy forest is worth far more than an acre of grass with a cow on it.

For those who do worry about what will happen to "all those cows," keep in mind that "all those cows" exist because man creates them by the millions every year. As people cease eating the flesh of cows, fewer animals will be bred. Horses did not disappear when automobiles took over the roads.

Our government is beginning to recognize the changing trends of scientific thought. Leading nutritionists and physicians are reversing their traditional support of the meat-laden diet. Television, radio, magazines, and other media, dispense nutritional advice advocating a great reduction in the consumption of saturated fats, found predominantly in flesh foods.[44]

A recognized and well-planned change of our national food habits does not have to produce great economic or personal inconvenience. Indeed, new opportunities would appear for many people. With the appropriate use of the media, including television specials, public service announcements, celebrity, endorsements, etc., the public could be educated and motivated to begin to adopt more ecologically sound dietary and lifestyle choices.

An enlightened government would help farmers and ranchers transition into more beneficial work and use of the land, without great personal or economic upheaval, it would encourage more imaginative agricultural projects, like forest fuel or fiber, or perhaps the generation of electricity from solar panels and wind turbines. A wise government would offer creative and accessible programs for low interest loans to purchase new farming equipment and modernize facilities.

Technical support and retraining programs could help traditional meat and dairy-producing people to create appropriate goods and services, in harmony with the needs of the public health, the economy, and the ecology. Those who wish to move to cities or otherwise leave farming and ranching, could be helped with subsidized home purchase loans, vocational school and college tuition grants, and other aids to help make less stressful their movement towards new livelihoods.

Such helpful "transition" programs to enable people to acquire new skills and security - plus the financing of solar panels to provide inexpensive electrical power and hot water for every household in the nation - could be funded by the government for the same amount of money spent by the United States military on weapons every 180 days.[44a]

Anything less than a far-seeing program of well-crafted societal change will create strains that will be felt by the entire nation, and the world. There is still time to heal ourselves and our planet. We must, however, look at current realities - an exploding population and the crushing technologic demands upon the Earth's life support systems by six billion humans. All our ecologic, political, and social problems are multiplied in magnitude by devoting huge amounts of land, water and energy, to create an animal-based diet. Fortunately, so many ecologic problems are improved or remedied as we evolve our food choices, as individuals and nations, towards plant-based nutrition.

I feel that vegan nutrition holds the key to raising healthy children, nourishing strong adults, and creating a brighter future for all of us. Your effort to increase your appreciation of vegan cuisine as the "best fuel for the human body" will be rewarded, whether you are a grown adult - in good health or striving to overcome an illness - a growing child, or someone who just loves good food.

For everyone who realizes "you are what you eat" (as well as "**who** you eat" - and what **they** ate!), welcome to the delicious world of vegan nutrition.

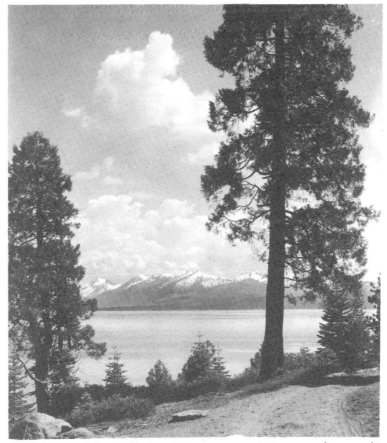

"We do not inherit the land from our ancestors, we borrow it from our children."

JOHN ROBBINS

PART TWO

WHAT NOT, WHY NOT

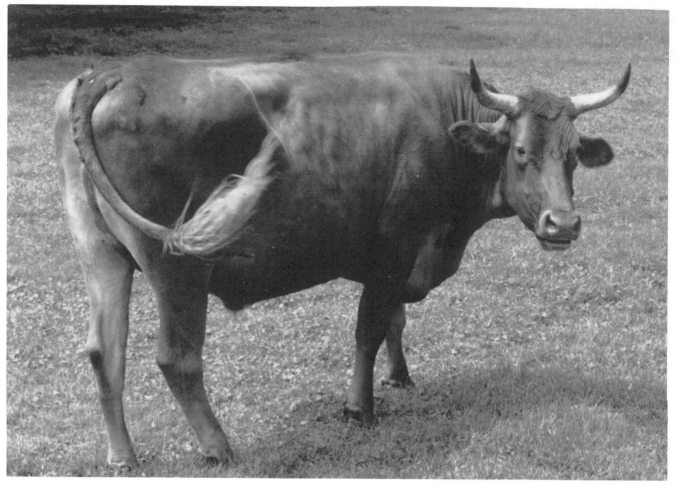

JUDY SUMMERS

CHAPTER FIVE

RED MEAT "BLUES"

The juicy T-bone steak and rare filet mignon, have long been viewed as "luxurious heights" of human nutrition. Red meat has traditionally been associated with strength, sensuality, and affluence. These beliefs are instilled in us from the first mouthful of meat chewed in childhood, with parents smiling approvingly. This early encouragement at the dinner table has been extremely effective.

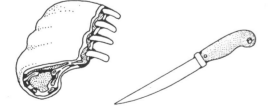

Consider for a moment how much animal flesh Americans consume in a lifetime. The average meat-eating American will eat:

    21 cows,
    14 sheep,
    12 hogs,
    900 chickens, and
    1,000 pounds of other animals, that either swam in the ocean, or flew in the air.[45]

These creatures are raised, fattened, and killed, not for human nutritional **requirements**, but rather, to supply a taste and chewing sensation that we acquired in childhood.

Animal muscle tissue disappears down American throats by the metric ton each year.

The reality is that "steak" is a piece of the leg muscle of a huge dead animal.

"Filet mignon" is really a cut of a long, thick muscle running deep in the cow's back along the lower spine.

"Shoulder cuts" are actually cuts of shoulder muscles, and "ribs" are the intercostal breathing muscles that move the pig's chest wall.

Prepared meats, like sausages and luncheon meats, such as bologna and hot dogs, often contain slaughterhouse scraps, like blood vessels, entrails, skin fragments, etc., which are ground up and homogenized to disguise their true identity.

To make matters worse, the cows, steers, lambs and pigs used for slaughter meat are fed **hormones and antibiotics**, the residues of which remain in active form in the steaks, burgers, and other meat products consumed by millions of Americans.[46] Cows drink water polluted with **heavy metals, pesticide residues, and radioactive isotopes**, which then appear in hot dogs and beefburgers.[47]

Additionally, all red meat contains **saturated fat.** The majority of this fat is the "marbling" mixed in with the muscle fibers. There is no such thing as truly lean meat. Trimming away the edge ring of fat around a steak really does not lower the fat content significantly. People who have red meat (trimmed or untrimmed) as a regular feature of their diets suffer in far greater numbers from heart attacks and strokes.[48]

A diet with fat-rich red meats also increases the risk of cancer - of the breast in women and of the prostate in men - most likely by upsetting delicately balanced levels of **sex and growth hormones.**

The body of a woman who eats animal fat will create high levels of the hormones, estrogen and prolactin, which stimulate the growth of breast tissue, the lining of the uterus, and many other tissues. It should come as no surprise that women who live with elevated levels of growth-promoting hormones in the blood flowing through their breast tissue, have higher rates of tumors and cancers of the breast and uterus.[49]

Correspondingly, men eating fatty meats are likely to have elevated levels of growth-stimulating androgens that increase the likelihood of developing cancer of the prostate gland.[50]

Eating red meats is also implicated as a cause of cancer of the colon. The probable reason for this is that when the cholesterol in meat is acted upon by bacteria in the colon, products are created that are powerful carcinogens. When beef is barbequed, the fat that drips into the fire is changed by the heat into benzopyrene, a potent carcinogen. This chemical then rises in the smoke and coats the surface of the steak, which is then eaten. In the intestine of the average meat-eating person, these substances are smeared against the bowel wall hour after hour, day after day.

As you might expect, colon cancer is epidemic in countries where large amounts of red meat are eaten,[51] and extremely rare in long-time vegans.[52] Predictably, ridding one's diet of red flesh, and changing to a vegan style of eating, greatly reduces one's risk of developing intestinal cancer.

Of course, the fat in red meat also contributes to obesity, and to all the obesity-related problems like diabetes, high blood pressure, degenerative arthritis, and gout. Fortunately, most of these problems improve or disappear as red meats in the diet yield to healthier staple items like pastas and potatoes.[53]

As will be further described in the chapters, "CHICKEN OUT," and "A FISHY STORY," the **concentrated protein** in all meats injures the kidney filters[54] contributing to kidney failure, and leaches calcium from the bones, leading to osteoporosis.[55]

Thus, the meat-laden, Western style diet, rather than leading us to an age of prosperity and health, has contributed to an epidemic of degenerative diseases. The nations who consume the most red meats suffer the highest rates of death from heart attacks, strokes, cancer, and diabetes.[56]

In view of the profound adverse health consequences that stem from eating animal flesh, we must seriously consider the explanation that Homo sapiens simply has not evolved into a carnivorous animal. Unlike the tiger, human beings do not have long, overlapping fangs, hinged jaws, short intestines, or a hunger for raw, freshly killed, bloody flesh. We have small mouths, short, flat, grinding molar teeth, and long intestines for digesting plant fiber. Instead of flesh-tearing claws, we have deft fingers that can pick fruit and peel vegetables.

If you believe that we were designed to eat animal flesh, consider this thought exercise:

Imagine running up to the nearest cow or bull, jumping on its back, opening your mouth, and trying to sink your teeth into its haunches. What would be the reality of your situation? You would soon find that your human mouth is very small and that your teeth - even your canines - are very short. You would be unable to even bite through the cow's tough hide, let alone through its raw muscle.

Humans are not carnivorous by their anatomy, nor by their nature. If we were true carnivores, we would walk into a butcher shop, purchase a large slab of raw cow flesh, leave the store, sit down on the curb, tear off the wrapping paper, and devour the bloody flesh with gusto.

PHYSIOLOGICAL COMPARISONS

<u>Carnivore</u>	<u>Herbivore</u>	<u>Human</u>
has claws	no claws	no claws
no skin pores, perspires through tongue	perspires through skin pores	perspires through skin pores
sharp front teeth for tearing, no flat molar teeth for grinding	no sharp front teeth, has flat molar teeth for grinding	no sharp front teeth, has flat molar teeth for grinding
intestinal tract (3) times body length so rapidly decaying meat can pass out quickly	intestinal tract 10 -12 times body length	intestinal tract 12 times body length
strong hydrochloric acid in stomach to digest meat	stomach acid 20 times weaker than meat eaters	stomach acid 20 times weaker than meat eaters

This is a repugnant thought to most people. In fact, to make animal flesh palatable to humans, it generally must be changed beyond recognition. It is cooked, seasoned, smothered in ketchup, or otherwise altered to disguise its true nature - the muscle of a large, dead animal. Yet, the thought of eating a raw apple, watermelon, or salad is pleasing to most of us. Food for thought, yes?

The anatomy of the human digestive system is excellently "engineered" to digest plant-based "fuels", high in fiber and complex carbohydrates, and only moderate in protein. Freed from the fiberless, fatty burden of red meat (and other flesh), our digestive systems perform smoothly and efficiently.

The details of how to use non-animal foods in one's daily life are presented in PART THREE. For now, it is enough to see the hazards of red meat in the human diet, and begin to substitute non-meat entrees for lunches and dinners wherever possible. There is nothing in red meat essential for human strength or health that cannot be obtained from safer, healthier sources. And remember, world class body builder, Andres Cahling, marathon swimmer, Murray Rose, and thousands of other vegetarian athletes around the world will attest that you do not have to eat a bull to be as strong as one.

So, how about spaghetti with tomato/mushroom sauce tonight? The food suggestions in PART THREE will make your personal journey to healthier vegan nutrition easy and delicious.

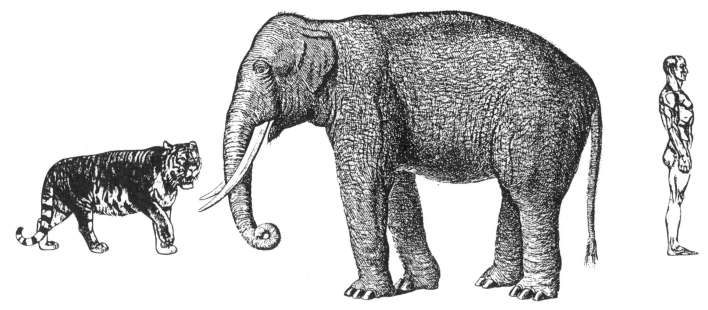

CHAPTER SIX

CHICKEN OUT!

For the past few years, Americans have been eating less beef and other red meats. This is a very good idea, for reasons that have already been presented in RED MEAT "BLUES". However, in their "stampede" away from beef, many Americans are turning to eating chickens, turkeys, ducks and other birds, for red meat substitutes.

This is ill-advised for the following reasons:

1. Although promoted for its low **fat** content, chicken flesh is not a very lean meat. White meat chicken (with skin) contains almost three teaspoons of chicken fat in every (small) three- ounce serving; chicken without the skin still packs 1.2 teaspoons of artery-clogging fat. [57] If you have ever seen chicken soup cooking in the pot, you have seen the fatty truth of chicken flesh in the oily, yellow globules floating on the water. Chicken fat, like all animal fat, spells trouble in your bloodstream.

2. People who consume large amounts of meat protein, like chicken flesh, are more susceptible to thin, easily fracturing bones, a condition known as **osteoporosis.** (See "A FISHY STORY," next). The more protein in the diet, the greater the calcium loss from the body's bones, out through the kidneys. As you might expect, osteoporosis is most rampant in the countries which consume the most poultry and other meats. [58]

3 The increasing **salmonella bacterial contamination** of chicken is a severe threat to the public health. Infection from this bacteria can cause severe dehydrating diarrhea, infection of lungs and nervous system, a linger arthritis, and not infrequently, death. The U.S. Communicable Disease Center and the Food and Drug Administration estimates that in 1985, four million Americans became infected with salmonella bacteria.[60] Thirty-five thousand people were hospitalized. One hundred twenty thousand victims were left with chronic, crippling arthritis, and 1,000 people died.

The cost in hospital expenses, lost work time and human suffering due to salmonella poisoning from poultry is staggering. Millions of cases of the "flu" that strike people each year are suspected as being salmonella food poisoning. Poultry is the prime carrier of this bacteria to American dinner tables. [61]

Salmonella contamination is endemic in the poultry industry. This chronic contamination largely results from feeding grain to chickens that is laced with antibiotics and mixed with salmonella-tainted chicken manure as a "volume extender" and protein "booster". (Such bacterially-tainted volume extenders made with chicken manure are also fed to cattle, thus promoting the spread of Salmonella to beef products as well.) According to the U. S. Department of Agriculture's own inspection records, at least one out of three chickens purchased at the supermarket is contaminated with salmonella bacteria.

The very act of cutting and preparing such a bird carcass will almost surely contaminate the kitchen counter, cutting boards, knives and other utensils, and "clean-up" sponges. A contaminated knife used to cut vegetables, or a salmonella- tainted spoon dipped into the potato salad, would quickly spread the contamination to other foods prepared in the same kitchen. This seems like reason enough to abstain from bringing these contaminated carcasses into the kitchen where food is prepared.

4. There is a disturbing relationship between chickens and **lymphoma,** cancer of the lymph nodes. Lymphoma is the most common cancer of chickens, and is caused by a virus passed from chicken to chicken. It is called "Marek's disease," and there is a strong suspicion that this virus can induce cancer of the lymph nodes in people.[62]

Poultry farmers have an alarmingly high rate of lymph cancer of any occupation.[63] They work in chicken houses, breathing the dust, and, of course, most eat a lot of chicken meat. Medical researchers who have worked with the chicken lymphoma viruses have contracted cancers of their own lymph nodes and the tumors of humans and chickens are almost indistinguishable.[64]

Linking chicken to these cancer viruses has yet to be conclusively proven, but the evidence of the connection is quite worrisome.[65]

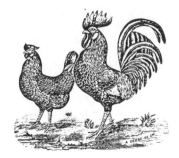

6. Before we "fly the coop," let's consider another health- threatening product taken from chickens, their **eggs**:

Eggs carry a triple load of trouble for people who eat them:

(a) **The yolk of a hen's egg is one the densest concentrations of animal fat on the planet.** It is made to fuel a baby chicken for twenty-one days with no other energy. When egg yolks are eaten, this concentrated fat pours through the bloodstream, raising the cholesterol and thus contributing to clogging of the arteries. [66]

(b) The **albumin protein** of egg whites is very concentrated, and, like all concentrated animal proteins, can contribute to leaching calcium out of the bones, leading to osteoporosis. [67]

(c) Egg products have been shown to be carriers of **salmonella bacteria**, with all the problems that implies. The salmonella bacteria populates the chicken's egg-producing organs, and thus contaminate the egg from within, before the shell goes on. [68]

There is no reason why a healthy human being should eat the eggs of chickens, and very good reasons why not.

Rather than ingesting chicken meat, eggs, and other poultry products, the wise consumer, seeking "clean protein," should rely on tofu, legumes, grains, green vegetables, and other nutritious non-animal foods. The tastes of delicious vegan dishes, like grain-burgers, tofu cutlets, seitan stew, and tempeh creations, soon replace the desires for the muscles of chickens, turkeys, ducks, geese, Cornish hens, and other commonly eaten birds. Here is one time when "chickening out" is a brave move, and a smart one, too.

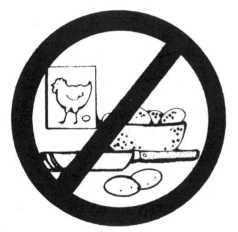

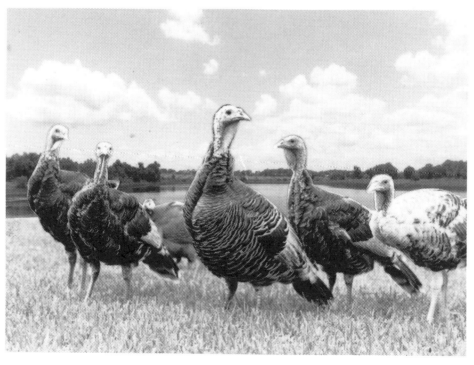

JUDY SUMMERS

CHAPTER SEVEN

A FISHY STORY

Until recently, fish has been advocated as a healthy substitute for meat in the diet. Before getting hooked by that idea, consider this:

EATING FISH FLESH, OR FISH BY-PRODUCTS, IS HAZARDOUS TO HUMAN HEALTH

1. FISH FLESH AND FISH OIL CONTAIN TOXIC CHEMICAL POLLUTANTS

The toxic wastes from 20th Century society are poured into rivers and oceans and become incorporated into the biosystem. These poisons concentrate in the flesh of the fish who eat "at the top of the food chain". Fish flesh regularly contains toxic chemical pollutants known to cause cancer, kidney failure, nerve damage, and birth defects. Much (most?) fish flesh has been shown to harbor large amounts of any or all of the following:

Heavy metals from industrial wastes. Arsenic, methylmercury, aluminum, cadmium, etc., [69] are flushed into streams and rivers, and washed into the bays and oceans to be taken up by the free-swimming fish and bottom dwellers (oysters, crabs, clams, mussels, scallops, flounders, lobsters, shrimp, etc.)

Mutation-inducing Hydrocarbons. Mutagenic polychlorinated biphenyls (PCB's), hydrocarbon pesticides, herbicides, dioxins, etc., from spraying of crops wash down from the fields, through the rivers and streams, and finally out into the ocean where they find their way into the bodies of free-swimming and bottom dwelling fish.[70]

Radioactivity from nuclear pollution.[71] Most nuclear power plants are built along rivers, so that water may be used to cool the reactor. Accidents in nuclear power plants and waste spillage from transport trucks, pipe leakage, etc, can result in radioactive contamination of the nearby waterway and the animals who make it their home.

Few U.S. waters (and indeed, world waters) are free of hydrocarbon or heavy metal pollution; this includes open sea waters, as well as most of our streams, lakes and rivers. As one might expect from living in waters laced with carcinogenic chemicals, the fish themselves show alarmingly high rates of cancer. The medical literature is filled with reports of toxicity of these chemicals to fish and to the people who eat them.

Here are some examples worth considering:

Pollutants such as PCB's, DDT, and dioxin, concentrate in the muscle tissue of fish. Eating a one-pound fish from Lake Ontario is equivalent to drinking 1.5 million quarts of that polluted water.[72]

Up to 80% of pike and other fish taken from lakes and rivers in New York State, Ohio, and Michigan, suffer from obvious cancerous tumors of skin and liver. Carcinogenic hydrocarbons concentrate to high levels in bottom-feeding fish in rivers in Maryland,[73] in the Nile in Egypt,[74] and in the Apalachicola River in Florida.[75] There are also alarming reports of carcinogenic residues in the fish taken from the open ocean, like the Mediterranean[76] and Baltic Seas.[77]

These pollutants exert serious toxic effects upon all aquatic animals, but especially upon those animals that feed on the bottom of rivers, lakes and oceans, where chemicals concentrate and enter the animals' food chain. Oysters, clams, and mussels have all been found with excessive levels of pollutants[78]. As filter feeders, they eliminate contaminants through their feces. People usually eat clams and oysters whole, and so, humans consume not only the toxins concentrated in the animal's tissues, but also those trapped in the fecal matter left in the intestinal tract. In Monterey, California, mussels found in 1984 had lead contamination 150 times greater than the maximum level determined "fit" for human consumption.

Consumers have little way of knowing where the fish they buy comes from, **or where it has been**. There is virtually no government quality or safety inspection of fish or fish products. Less than 13% of fish are inspected by any government agency.[79]

Numerous (and increasing numbers of) medical studies describe signs of **poisoning in people** that seem to result from eating contaminated fish. The following examples illustrate this health threat:

A. Nerve toxicity from methylmercury poisoning and increased rates of some cancers are seen in Japanese people who eat fish.[80]

B. The Mohawk Indians tested in New York, and the natives of Lake Murray, New Guinea, showed signs of nerve damage as well as elevated levels of mercury in their blood and tissues.[81]

C. Canadian Indians in northern Quebec have suffered numerous incidents of kidney damage from methylmercury poisoning after eating mercury- contaminated fish.[82]

D. Finnish children who eat fish have increased intakes of mercury, lead, cadmium, and arsenic.[83]

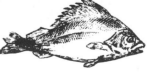

E. German citizens living along the River Elbe, in Schleswig-Holstein, as well as the fish from the river, have higher levels of organochlorines and mercury in their blood.[84]

F. Uranium radionuclides permeate the food chain in northern Saskatchewan. [85]

G. Lead accumulates to high levels in the fish in the Missouri River downstream of the lead mines. [86]

H. Breastfeeding women who eat fish show significant levels of DDT and other pesticides in the breast milk they feed to their infants. [87]

Fish flesh decomposes more rapidly and with a more foul odor than any other type of meat. On board the fishing ship, the weight of the fish in the hold crushes the bottommost animals, often forcing their intestinal contents out and causing contamination. In their attempt to retard the spoilage, fishermen spray the dying fish in the hold of their ships with antibiotic solutions or ice containing antibiotics (often made from the polluted waters in which they have been fishing).

When considering eating a piece of a fish, stop and ask yourself, "What's in it today?" The human body has no requirement for their flesh and certainly has no need for the contaminants listed above.

2. FISH EATING IS LINKED WITH OSTEOPOROSIS

Fish flesh is **very** concentrated protein. Protein cannot be stored, and any protein eaten over the amount that can be used on a given day is broken down and excreted. After all, you can only make so much blood and grow so much hair each day.

Only 20 to 30 grams of protein are needed by your body each day.[88] A large piece of fish flesh and a glass of milk can contain 100 grams (or more) of protein. After eating any concentrated protein, like a fish fillet or halibut steak, the kidneys must cleanse the blood of protein wastes like ammonia, urea, amino acid fragments, etc.

The kidneys do oblige, of course, but to accomplish this blood cleansing, there is a predictable loss of calcium following the ingestion of concentrated protein.

This means that for hours after eating a piece of fish, precious calcium pours out of your body with each urination. This is a well-known and reproducable phenomenon called, **"protein-induced hypercalcuria,"**[89]--and the calcium that is leaving the blood is really being taken out of the body's vital storehouse of calcium, the bones.

This calcium loss, continued year after year, drains calcium from the skeleton, resulting in thin, crumbly bones that fracture easily, called **osteoporosis.** This condition affects 15 million Americans, and is not so much a disease of calcium deficiency, but rather, a **disease of protein excess**. Osteoporosis is most severe in the people who consume the most protein [90] and is most rampant among the Eskimos. These northern natives eat large quantities of fish in their diet - averaging 150 to 200 grams of protein daily - and still lose mineral from their skeleton, despite eating 2000 milligrams of calcium each day contained in fish bones. [91]

All the gently-absorbed protein needed for human health and growth is obtainable from the grains, legumes, greens, nuts and seeds found in a meat and dairy-free vegan diet. [92] These are far safer sources from which to obtain our protein. Vegetable protein is less prone to cause calcium loss due to its slower absorption and less acid nature.

3. HAZARDS OF FISH OIL AS A DIETARY SUPPLEMENT

Recently, fish oil has been trumpeted as a protective substance against clogged arteries and heart attacks. The much heralded "advantages" from consuming fish products are overshadowed by the hazards of eating fish flesh or the oil extracted from the fish's liver. The fish oils that are promoted as providing protection to the arteries from atherosclerosis may also pose a serious hazard because they **decrease the blood's ability to coagulate to stop bleeding.**

Eskimos, who eat large amounts of fish, suffer high rates of hemorrhagic strokes, nose bleeds, and epilepsy. [93] This "blood thinning" property could be exceedingly dangerous for anyone suffering a stroke, which would occur when a blood vessel in the brain bursts, and the blood fails to clot.

Fish oil has also been shown to **inhibit the action of insulin.** This is bad news for any diabetic trying to maintain normal blood sugar levels while eating a diet high in fish flesh. Diabetics achieve much better control of their condition on a high-fiber, plant-based diet.

An unpublicized, but potentially important problem results from fish oil's apparent tendency to **increase the length of a normal pregnancy.** An overly long gestation time increases the birthweight of the baby, and thus the attendant risk of birth accidents, cesarean sections, and maternal deaths. Birthweights in the Faroe Islands (in the North Atlantic), where the people eat a large amount of fish oils, are among the highest in the world. As might be expected, death rates during late pregnancy are twice as high in the Faroe Islands as they are in Denmark, which has a much lower consumption of fish oil. [94]

Excessive consumption of all oils, including fish oil, is linked to increased cancer growth [95], and contributes to gallbladder disease. [96]

Despite current advertising campaigns, no one needs to eat the oil squeezed out of a fish's flesh or liver; in fact, the products of a fish's liver, as in cod liver oil, is one of the strangest substances to consider eating. The liver of any animal is the chemical detoxifier for the body, and thus concentrates all the pollutants consumed by that animal. The oil squeezed from fish livers contains high levels of the toxins listed above, plus large amounts of cholesterol. A single fish oil capsule can contain 300 milligrams of cholesterol, yet the body can only excrete 100 milligrams of that greasy substance each day. Fish oil is a substance whose potential problems outweigh its possible benefits to health.

Fish oil capsules are not "magic pills" that will allow people to continue eating fatty meats and dairy products without clogging their arteries. People who use fish oil "to protect their arteries" may actually be poisoning themselves with heavy metals and hydrocarbons, and increasing their cancer risk from dietary oils. The better solution is to keep one's arteries clean, by not loading the blood with animal fat in the first place. People who do not eat animal fats generally do not suffer from clogged arteries, and thus have no need to eat the oil of fish.

The human body has a need for essential oils, but vegetarians can take heart (so to speak) because the "good" in oils sought from fish sources are available in vegetarian foods. "EPA" (eicosapentaenoic acid - one of the "fat lowering" oils sought in fish products) is found in walnuts, wheat germ oil, soybean lecithin, flaxseed oil [97], soybeans and tofu, common beans, and seaweed.

LET THEM SWIM. . .

In conclusion, (a) the carcinogenic and nerve-damaging chemical contaminants, (b) the calcium-robbing protein load, and (c) the potentially hazardous, blood-altering oils, make the idea of eating fresh water or marine animals a "fishy" one. Fish is **not** "brain food" - in fact, it is just the opposite: mercury poisons the brain and nerve cells.

Because a vegan diet meets **all** the human body's nutritional needs, and naturally offers protection against clogged arteries, heart attacks, strokes and cancers, [98] you will do your health (and the fish!) a favor by letting them "off the hook".

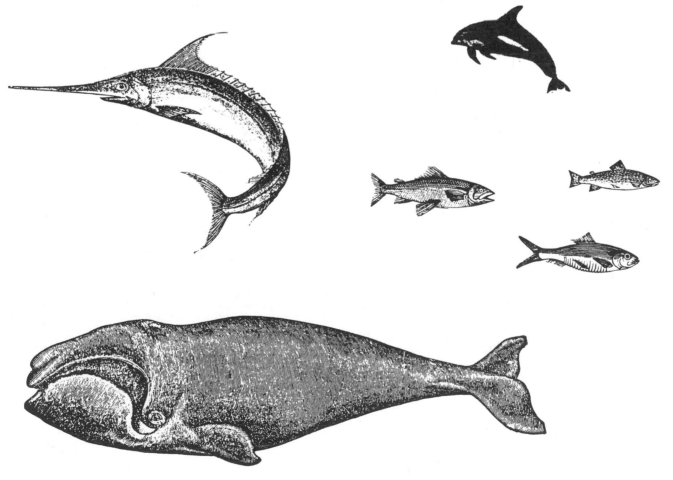

CHAPTER 8

NOW HOW, BROWN COW?

Our "rogues' gallery" of health-destroying animal products would not be complete without considering the white fluid drawn from the udders of cows. There are many problems associated with milk and products made from it.

Cow's milk is a superbly designed, high-fat fluid designed by Nature to turn a 65-pound calf into a 600-pound cow in six months. It has a "bovine" mixture of casein protein and saturated fat, and simply is not a natural food for man, woman or child.

Milk was never meant to see the light of day; it is the mother's flowing gift of life to her newborn baby - human, calf or other mammal - and is meant to flow directly from the mother's nipple to the baby's lips. The dairy farm operation is a grim distortion of this process.

Cows are artifically impregnated most every year, and give birth to calves that are almost immediately taken away from them. Female calves are added to the milking herd, while male calves are destined for sixteen weeks in a tiny wooden crate, chained by the neck, drinking iron-poor antibiotic-laced milk, to make them anemic, until their throats are cut and they are made into "milk-fed" veal.

The milk intended for the baby calf is sucked from the cow twice daily by a machine, pooled with other milk, and shipped to the dairy. There, the butterfat (cream) is separated from the milk, concentrated, and processed, and then sold to the public in various forms:

The butterfat is churned with air into BUTTER, or diluted with milk and sold as CREAM.

The butterfat/milk mixture is mixed with sugar, frozen, and sold as ICE CREAM.

The butterfat/milk mixture is congealed with rennet (from calf stomach) and bacteria, and then aged with fungus mold until it congeals into thick lumps, called CHEESE.

The buttterfat/milk mixture is fermented with bacteria into SOUR CREAM or YOGURT.

The butterfat is mixed with cocoa powder and sugar and sold as MILK CHOCOLATE.

These are all artery-clogging forms of animal fat made from cows milk.

Consider the fat content of these popular dairy foods:

Butter = 80%
Cream = 40%
Ice Cream = 20% - 40%
("Luxury" ice creams have the highest fat content.)
Cheese = 25% - 40%
Chocolate = 25% - 40%

Eating foods that contain these amounts and types of animal fats has been conclusively linked with heart attacks, strokes, and cancer growth. [99]

Dairy products also contain animal proteins, like casein, that can contribute to **allergic/inflammatory reactions,** such as chronic runny noses, recurrent ear and bronchial infections, eczema, asthmatic bronchitis[100], and other inflammations of joints [101], skin and bowels. [102]

COW'S MILK for CALCIUM? - A "MOOOOT" POINT

Although promoted as good sources of calcium, vital for strong bones, and "preventatives" against osteoporosis, milk, cheese, yogurt, and ice cream are not really wholesome sources of calcium. These dairy products contain significant amounts of **saturated fat, allergy-inciting cow protein,** and **pesticides,** as well as a large load of **phosphate,** which can neutralize the benefits of calcium.

Consuming dairy products does not seem to prevent osteoporosis. The nations with the highest levels of dairy product consumption are also the nations with the highest rates of osteoporosis [103]. This effect is probably due to the calcium-robbing effect of the accompanying concentrated protein load of animal products, **including the protein found in dairy products themselves.**

In one study, (sponsored by the Dairy Council!) women consuming three eight-ounce glasses of cow's milk per day still lost calcium from their bodies, and remained in negative calcium balance, even after a year of consuming almost fifteen hundred milligrams of calcium daily! [104] It is the high protein diet, laden with poultry, fish, and dairy products, that steals calcium from the body, rather than insufficient calcium consumed in the diet. [105] Taking extra calcium in the form of supplements has not been shown to be effective in preventing or reversing osteoporosis. [106] Any adult already experiencing osteoporosis, or feeling that they may be at risk for it, **can slow down the rate of calcium loss** from their body by:

1) adopting a healthful, **low-protein diet**

2) **stopping smoking**, as well as using **caffeine** and **acid soft drinks,** all of which rob calcium from the bones, and

3) taking a brisk 20 to 30-minute **walk** outside in the **sunshine** everyday.

Rather than making the calcium tablet-makers wealthy while trying to ward off osteoporosis, a solution is offered through good nutrition. The proteins in plant-based vegan foods are naturally less concentrated, and because they are mixed with oils and complex carbohydrates, are more slowly absorbed by the intestine. They do not flood the bloodstream with acid-forming protein, as happens after eating a piece of chicken muscle or drinking cow's milk. Calcium does not pour out of the body after a meal of spaghetti with tomato sauce, whole grain garlic bread, garden green salad, and steamed broccoli with mushroom gravy, as it does after eating a piece of fish or drinking a glass of milk.[107]

If dairy products do not belong in the human diet, where do we get our calcium and protein? Remember that pure vegetarian animals like buffalos and thoroughbred horses, create **huge** bone structures with hundreds of pounds of calcium and **never** drink milk or eat cheese. These magnificent (vegan) animals seem to know that calcium abounds in greens, grains, legumes, nuts, seeds, and vegetables - which is where we can obtain ours.

The United States Recommended Daily Allowance for calcium for non pregnant adults is 800 milligrams. The meals in the sample menu plan will provide at least this amount, completely free of dairy products and the contaminants they contain.

Dairy products also harbor a little-discussed, but very ominous connection with **leukemia** in children. As any veterinarian will verify, leukemia is common in dairy cows and is caused by a virus, bovine leukemia virus. A cow with leukemia passes this virus into the milk.[108] Up to 20% of the cows in a herd may be infected with leukemia virus. Their virus-laden milk is mixed with other milk and sold in stores.[109] Could the high rate of leukemia in children be connected to their high levels of milk consumption? Denmark, the country with the highest rate of leukemia in their cattle and in their children, has an active program to remove leukemic cows from the dairy herd.[110]

In view of the fact that we do not need cow's milk products for good health (the evidence suggests the opposite is true), its seems that the continued use of dairy products is largely to satisfy a national addiction to fats and sugars. Cow's milk is fit food only for baby calves. As physician and nutritionist John McDougall, M.D., states, "Pour cow's milk on your cereal? Why not dog's milk? Or horse's milk? They make just as much sense!

Fortunately, there are delicious and healthy alternatives to milk and dairy products, as listed in Appendix IV. Vanilla soymilk on cereal, banana "nice-cream malteds" for treats, and tofu "sour cream" on baked potatoes, easily replace the fatty foes from the dairy case. Again, no hardship is required, but rather, a journey of taste delights awaits your big "moooove."

Look past the advertising that bombards us, and see milk, cheese, ice cream, yogurt, butter, sour cream, and other dairy products, for the fatty health threats that they are. Most of the people on planet Earth live healthily without cow's milk products, and so can you.

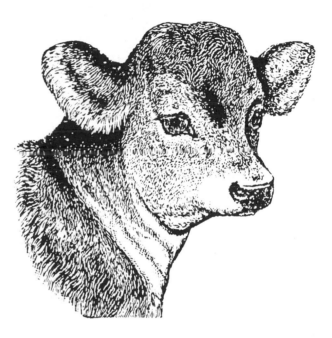

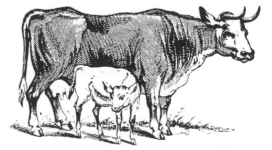

PART THREE

FOOD FOR A LIFETIME

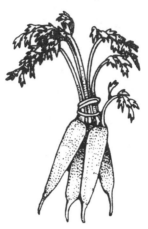

CHAPTER 9

BASIC TRAINING

In PART TWO we examined what not to eat, and why there is no such thing as "a good steak," or a "nutritious glass of milk." Before you despair that "there is nothing left to eat but lettuce and raisins," take heart - delicious food is on its way.

But first, let's consider some of the nutritional realities of the miracle you walk around in every day - your human body.

As stated in PART ONE, the simple fact is that:

**THE HUMAN BODY HAS NO NUTRITIONAL REQUIREMENT
FOR THE FLESH OR MILK OF ANIMALS.**

There is no nutrient essential for human health in animal flesh or cow's milk that cannot be obtained from plant-derived sources.

Some basic nutritional principles will make this clear. Daily body function for everyone, adult or child, pregnant or not, requires adequate intake of the following "Essential Six" basic nutrients. Give your body sufficient amounts of these nutritional cornerstones, and you will be well-nourished.

YOUR BODY'S "ESSENTIAL SIX"

First, our bodies need ENERGY (calories) to function. Humans derive their energy from:

(1). CARBOHYDRATES and (2.) OILS.

Like a car requires gasoline to run, so does the body require "fuel" for energy, to do its work of muscle contraction, nerve impulse conduction, hormone production, wound repair, cell growth, etc. This "cell fuel" is composed of the carbohydrates and oils made by plants, from sunlight, air and water, and it appears in the vegan diet as sugars, starches and vegetable oils. These fuels are found in abundance in **grains, vegetables, nuts, cooking oils, fruits,** etc.; it's easy for everyone to obtain enough each day if they enjoy their pastas, potatoes and fruit smoothies - and they're **not** fattening.

(3.) WATER

Pure water is needed so that the blood flows, the glands secrete vital fluids, and the chemical reactions of life can occur in the cells. We should try to drink at least three to six eight-ounce glasses per day in the form of pure **water, herbal teas, fruit juices, or vegetable juices.** We will obtain the balance of water needed (2 to 3 quarts daily) in the watery fruits, vegetables, soups, and salads that abound in vegan cuisine.

(4.) VITAMINS

Vitamins are necessary "co-workers" for the cells' enzymes ("the machinery") to perform their work of protein production and metabolism. Vitamins are to the cell enzymes as the oil and lubricating fluids in your car's engine are to the moving parts.

There are two types of vitamins:

a) **Water -Soluble Vitamins**: These are not stored in the body, and the supply must be renewed each day. Vitamin C, B-complex, folic acid, etc., are found in **green, leafy vegetables,** like collards, kale and broccoli, spinach, as well as citrus fruits and nutritional yeast. Enjoy fresh garden salads and steamed greens!

b) **Oil Soluble- Vitamins**: Vitamins like A, E, etc., are stored in the liver, and eating **yellow vegetables** several times per week is sufficient to meet all requirements. The richest supply of these vitamins are found in carrots, squash, and sweet potatoes; also found in dark greens like kale and broccoli, as well as in melons, like cantaloupe.

(5.) MINERALS

Minerals are Earth elements necessary for electrical and chemical reactions in the body cells. Potassium, iron, zinc, selenium, iodine, calcium, etc., are abundant in **green, leafy vegetables, grains, mushrooms, nutritional yeast, and sea vegetables** (arame, kombu, kelp, dulse, etc.)

(6.) PROTEIN

Protein is the "building block" material for making muscles, blood, hormones, new tissue, (hair, fingernails, skin, etc.), wound healing, bone growth, hormone production, immune antibodies, and in the case of pregnancy, the baby. **Grains, legumes, green vegetables, and nuts and seeds**, are excellent sources of protein, and can supply all the body's needs (See "A Closer Look at Protein").

That's it. Give the body sufficient amounts of these essential six nutrients, along with pleasant daily walks in the sunshine, clean air to breathe, and a low-stress lifestyle with generous amounts of laughter, and that body will grow strong and healthy.

A MATTER OF BALANCE. . .

Medical researchers are realizing that remarkable changes occur in the body when the tides of animal fats cease washing through the bloodstream.

When meat and dairy products are deleted from the diet, calories should be replaced by increased portions of grains and nuts, and the protein is replaced through increased portions of grains, legumes, and seeds.

When a "pure carbohydrate fuel" is given to the body, the balance of fats changes **everywhere.** The circulating fat levels in the bloodstreams of vegans are substantially lower than those of meat-eating people[111]. The vegan's balance of "good" fats versus "bad" fats (HDL/LDL ratio) is more favorable. As you might expect, this dramatically decreases their risk for heart attack and strokes.[112]

As mentioned, the favorable potassium/sodium balance of plant foods versus animal flesh is far more health promoting to the human body than the great sodium loads typical of a meat- based diet. Vegans generally run delightfully normal blood pressures, and thus are at much lower risk for strokes. A change to vegan nutrition can be a key factor in resolving a life-threatening problem of chronic high blood pressure.[113]

The normal state of health for the body is one of balance. The meat-laden American diet, that sends jolts of fat, protein, and salt through the arteries every few hours, is a powerful unbalancing force. However, a diet composed only of broccoli and apples, although vegan, could not be called balanced, either. Adequate amounts of protein, vitamins, minerals, and other essential nutrients are obtained through consuming the many varieties of food offered from the plant kingdom. When meat and dairy products are deleted, protein and calcium are replaced by increased use of green, leafy vegetables, legumes, nuts, and dried fruits, as well as fortified soy milks.

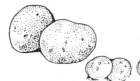

"THE VEGAN SIX" FOOD GROUPS

---

1. WHOLE GRAINS and POTATOES   4. NUTS and SEEDS

2. LEGUMES   5. FRUITS

3. GREEN and YELLOW VEGETABLES   6. VITAMIN and MINERAL FOODS

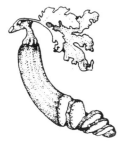

All the nutritional requirements for human health that were just presented can be conveniently (and safely) met by consuming ample portions each day from the "food families" of the "Vegan Six" Food Groups that follow. **"Balance"** in the vegan diet, that is, sufficient amounts of all the essential nutrients, is achieved by eating an appropriate number of servings from **each** group of the "Vegan Six" each day.

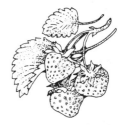

1. WHOLE GRAINS and STARCHES - including GRAIN PRODUCTS and POTATOES - Whole grain brown rice, corn, millet, barley, bulghur, buckwheat groats, oats (including oatmeal, granola, and other cereals), wheat (including cereals, breads, pastas, flour, etc.), amaranth, triticale, quinoa.

   Nutrients - Energy, protein, oils, vitamins, and fiber (for normal bowel function).

   Quantity - 2 - 4 (four-ounce) servings daily.

2. LEGUMES - (Anything that grows in a pod) - Green peas, lentils, chick peas (garbanzos), beans of all types (navy, lima, kidney, aduki, black beans, etc.), soybeans and soy products (soy milk, tofu, texturized vegetable protein granules, tempeh, etc.), peanuts, and **sprouted** seeds and legumes, such as alfalfa and mung bean sprouts.

   Nutrients - Protein and oils.

   Quantity - 1 - 2 (three - four ounce) serving daily.

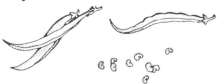

3. GREEN AND YELLOW VEGETABLES

   Green - Broccoli, collards, kale, brussels sprouts, spinach, swiss chard, cabbage, romaine, cucumbers, mustard greens, endive, etc.

   Yellow - Carrots, squash (acorn, butternut, hubbard, summer, spaghetti, etc.), sweet potatoes, pumpkins, parsnips, etc.

   Nutrients - Vitamins, minerals, protein

   Quantity - 1 - 2 (four-ounce) servings daily of greens, and 1 or 2 (four ounce) servings every other day for yellows.

4. NUTS AND SEEDS - Almonds, walnuts, pecans, cashews, filberts, macadamia, and nut butters made from these.

   Sesame seeds (and tahini butter made from them), sunflower seeds, and pumpkin seeds.

   Nutrients - Protein, oils, calcium, trace minerals

   Quantity - 1-3 (one-ounce) servings daily.

5. FRUITS of all kinds, especially citrus and melons.

Nutrients - Energy, vitamins and minerals.

Quantity - 3-6 servings daily.

6. VITAMIN B-12 AND MINERAL FOODS -
For trace minerals and vitamin B-12.

MINERAL FOODS

(a) Root vegetables - Carrots, beets, turnips, etc., as well as mushrooms,

and

(b) Sea vegetables - Arame, kombu, kelp, nori, spirulina, dulse, etc., are good sources of essential trace minerals, like iodine, manganese, copper, etc.

(c) A reliable source of Vitamin B-12 must be included in a balanced vegan diet. (See "Vitamin B-12" section for description of available B-12 sources)

NOTE: **Nutritional yeast** and **fermented soy products,** like tempeh, unless specifically fortified, contain **variable** amounts of Vitamin B-12. Thus, they should not be relied upon as the **sole** source of Vitamin B-12 in a vegan diet.

Quantity - 1 serving of (a), (b), and (c), at least three times weekly.

There they are, the "VEGAN SIX" - all the foods you will ever need to eat to keep your body strong and healthy.

REAL FOOD FOR REAL (VEGAN) PEOPLE

Because the "Vegan Six" consists of wholesome ingredients with ample fresh fruits and vegetables, there are many tasty treasures awaiting you. Let's consider some examples of "real foods," and then look at some dishes made from the "Vegan Six" that supply the most important nutrients.

After a morning stretch and a walk, think about a healthy -

BREAKFAST

There are many ideas about what constitutes a good breakfast.

People who prefer to keep their morning food light and cleansing, can follow the "fruit till noon" guideline. They can enjoy individual pieces of melon, peaches, apples, bananas, and plums, or combine them all in a "fruit bowl," topped with fruit juice and shredded coconut. Fruit meals are especially refreshing on a hot day, and can be used as a lunch or dinner theme as well.

Some say about melons and citrus: "Eat them alone, or leave them alone." This may be good advice for some people. Each person must find out the truth of this for him or her self.

Fans of a more substantial breakfast will savor a stack of whole grain pancakes with real maple syrup, or strawberry (blueberry) jam.

HINT - On the pancakes, if melted butter was previously used, exchange it for a teaspoon of olive, flaxseed or safflower oil.

Former scrambled egg aficionados will delight in a golden tofu "omelette," Western style, with chopped red and green peppers and onions. It's easy to learn, quick to make, and cholesterol-free.

Baked, sliced plantains, with corn or bran muffins and fruit spread, create a carbohydrate and fiber-rich breakfast with a tropical flavor.

The cereal shelf at the supermarket and health food store offers many flaked cereals, as well as relatively unprocessed whole grains (rolled oats, rye flakes, etc.). Commercially processed cereals, although no longer in their "natural form," do contain some useful protein and fiber, and are usually fortified with Vitamin B-12, and thus they are a reasonable breakfast choice up to several times per week. On cold mornings, a bowl of hot oatmeal can be served with raisins, sunflower seeds, and a dash of cinnamon, and topped with fruit and sweet vanilla soymilk, or blender-made sunflower milk.

Whole grain toast, with peanut butter and fruit preserves, is a favorite "instant breakfast," high in protein and energy.

As mid-day arrives, it's time to think about -

LUNCH

Open your refrigerator or lunchbox and warm up the delicately seasoned "veggie-grain burger" on a whole wheat bun with lettuce, tomatoes, sprouts, and "all the trimmings." A fresh green salad with non-dairy French dressing and a thermos of last night's vegetable-bean soup balance the meal. A chocolatey carob brownie makes a sweet dessert.

(Other sandwich ideas include whole grain bread with peanut, almond, or cashew butter with fruit spread, or pita bread, filled with a chickpea hummus or tofu spread.)

A RELIABLE FORMULA FOR A BALANCED LUNCH (OR DINNER) IS:

<u>SALAD</u> - Fresh green Salad,

<u>ENTREE</u> - A grain/legume combination, ("2 1/2 to 1" grain to legume mix; that is 2 1/2 cups grain to 1 cup lentils, peas, beans, chickpeas, etc.)

<u>SIDE DISHES</u> - Serve yellow and/or green vegetables.

<u>DRESSING/SAUCE</u> - Topped by a nutrient-rich gravy, such as nutritional yeast /tahini, a tofu-based dressing, homemade tomato sauce, etc.

With the help of mid-afternoon fruit snacks, the day goes by quickly, and it is time to look forward to -

DINNER

A hearty, easy-to-make vegetable soup and/or green salad can again precede the entree.

Satisfying salads include: coleslaw, potato salad, raw carrot salad, spinach-mushroom, guacamole, cold bean salad, and tofu "egg-less" salad.

Full-bodied soups can feature: split pea, beet borscht, Scotch carrot/barley, tomato/gazpacho, vegetable/ bean, lentil, or hot miso with noodles.

The main dish entree, which is based upon grains and/or potatoes, can display the colorful and tasty vegetarian tradition from countries around the globe, such as these:

From Italy, enjoy Meatless Lasagna, Egg-plant   Milanese, or Spaghetti and Tofu Balls.

How about Oriental Stir-Fried Vegetables with Cashews served over rice or noodles?

An evening in "old Mexico" can begin with Corn Enchilladas or Tacos with Beans, or a spicy "Chili con Tofu."

A Mediterranean flavor can be created with Chickpea Hummus and chopped vegetables in whole wheat pocket pita bread.

Hearty Potato Kugel with greens, Stuffed Cabbage with gravy, and Tahini/Vegetable Bake, all lend an Old World flavor.

Of course, there are delicious sauces and gravies to add flavor to most every dish.

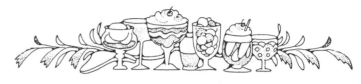

BEVERAGES

Healthful options for drinking include pure water, fresh fruit juices, herbal teas and coffee-style beverages, like Postum, Caffix, and Pero. Non-dairy soy or nut milks, and fruit smoothies can be enjoyed between meals or with snacks. (See "Dairy Alternatives," Appendix IV.)

SNACKS AND DESSERTS

Fresh fruits, eaten at least an hour after the main course, are satisfying and wholesome, as is popcorn, or raw nuts, like almonds, cashews, walnuts, and fil-berts.

For sweet desserts, versatile vegan cuisine offers many treats, like apple pie, carob cookies, Danish pastry, banana/raisin bread, tofu "cheesecake," as well as non-dairy "nice cream," yogurt, puddings, and candies.

Sample menus for two complete days of vegan meals, including numerical nutritional analyses, will soon be presented, showing that one can meet or exceed all the U. S. Recommended Daily Allowances (R.D.A.'s) on a balanced vegan diet.

People who are sensitive or have actual allergies to soy products, should substitute chickpeas, lentils, peas, or other legumes for soy foods such as tofu, tempeh, soy milk, etc.

People who are sensitive or have actual allergies to wheat, should choose pastas and breads made from rice, barley, or other grain flours.

THE "RIGHT STUFF"

Recall that the human digestive system, with its grinding molar teeth and long intestines, is ideally engineered to digest a plant-based diet. Herbivorous animals, who never take nutrition courses, and who also do not get high blood pressure, osteoporosis or clogged arteries, naturally eat a wide variety of plant foods, containing grains, legumes, greens, vegetables, and fruits. The good news is that the food formula that works so well for them, works for us, too!

People eating in the vegan style soon experience their bodies becoming more balanced, and they intuitively feel that animal-free foods are the best for them.

For those who desire reassurance "by the numbers," here are the nutritional "credentials" of the vegan diet.

THE NUMBERS GAME

Most nutritional concerns expressed about the vegan diet center on the requirements for **protein, calcium, iron**, and certain **vitamins**, such as **B-12, D,** and **folic acid**. Each of these will be considered individually. We'll begin by examining the current United States R.D.A.'s for these nutrients, and see how each of these needs can be conveniently and efficiently met with vegan food sources only.

The average non-pregnant adult requires each day:

PROTEIN: 56 grams for males
(the weight of 18 pennies)

44 grams for females
(the weight of 15 pennies)

CALCIUM: 800 milligrams

IRON: 10 milligrams for males
18 milligrams for females

VITAMIN B-12: 2-3 micrograms

VITAMIN D: 400 I.U.

FOLIC ACID: 5 milligrams

(For requirements and nutritional strategies for pregnant women and growing children, see the author's **PREGNANCY, CHILDREN, and THE VEGAN DIET**. In this work, we will concentrate upon the nutritional needs of adults.)

Let's first consider a topic dear to the heart of every vegetarian - PROTEIN.

I. PROTEIN

Much unnecessary worry has been generated over "getting enough protein". Two important facts must be kept in mind:

1. Too much protein is unhealthy, and **Americans eat too much protein!** The actual requirement to make new hair, blood and hormones, is only 20 to 40 grams of protein daily - about the weight of ten pennies [114]. The R.D.A.'s are intentionally set substantially higher than actual metabolic needs, to insure abundant intake in every case. Because of meat's concentrated protein loads, most people on the meat-laden American style diet eat an average protein load of 90 to 120 grams each day - the weight of 40 pennies! [115]

As mentioned in Chapter One, these excessive protein loads can cause damage to the kidneys by clogging the "filter units," leading to kidney failure [116], as well as contributing to osteoporosis. Meat-laden, high protein meals are no bargain for your health.

2. The idea of plant protein being "incomplete" and lacking some amino acids has been shown to be a myth. [117] Nature simply cannot make a soybean, potato, or grain of wheat without using **all** the same amino acids (the "building blocks" of protein) required by the metabolism of humans. [118] Rice, corn, potatoes, and wheat, have all been shown to keep people in positive protein balance when used as the sole protein source. [119] It is almost impossible to design a calorically adequate (2000 calorie) diet, utilizing foods from all the "Vegan Six" groups, and not obtain at least 50 grams of high-quality, "complete" protein.

Contrary to popular belief, it is **not necessary** to combine proteins at each meal. The protein from the whole grain toast enjoyed at breakfast, as well as the tofu in the dinner casserole, are "complete" in their own right, and will each find their way to your liver and other tissues and be well utilized. However, the more variety in protein sources, the better.

To assure yourself abundant protein while planning your lunch and dinner main dishes, accent the following "PROTEIN ALL-STARS" from the first four of the "VEGAN SIX".

PROTEIN ALL-STARS

GRAINS - Brown rice, oats (cereals - oatmeal, granola, etc.) millet, corn, barley, bulghur, wheat (including whole wheat bread, pastas, cereals, flour, etc.)

LEGUMES - Green peas, lentils, chick peas, alfalfa sprouts, mung beans, and beans of all kinds (kidney, lima, aduki, navy beans, soy beans and products made from them; e.g., tofu, texturized vegetable protein granules [TVP], tempeh, soy milks), peanuts, etc.

GREENS - Broccoli, collards, spinach, etc.

NUTS AND SEEDS - Almonds, cashews, walnuts, filberts, pistachios, pecans, macadamias and nut butters made from these.

Sunflower seeds, sesame seeds (including tahini butter made from ground sesame seeds), pumpkin seeds, etc.

Now that we've just learned that protein-rich foods do have high nutritional values when eaten separately, let it be said that **combining protein-rich ingredients does increase the protein absorption by about 30%, and thus variety is always a good strategy in vegan meal planning.**

So, to provide examples for help in meal planning (and not to cause worry about possible protein deficiency), here are some classic high-protein combinations from vegan cuisine. These protein-rich dishes will replace meat and dairy products in the human diet, while avoiding the burden of saturated fats and adulterants.

Two ample helpings of any of the following combinations average 15 to 35 grams of high-quality protein, and thus will provide a large measure of the daily protein requirements for a healthy adult.

SPROUTS

Sprouts are a wonderfully nutritious food source. They pack vitamins, minerals, and protein into a small volume, and have a fresh, live quality that seems to make humans healthier.

All seeds, grains, and legumes can (and many say should) be sprouted (or soaked overnight) before their use in meal preparation. **The soaking/sprouting**

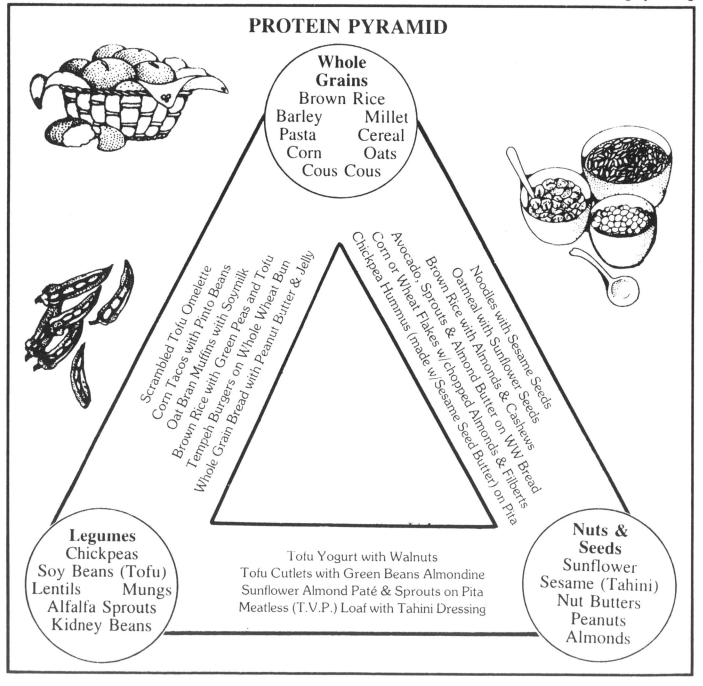

PROTEIN PYRAMID

Whole Grains
Brown Rice
Barley   Millet
Pasta   Cereal
Corn   Oats
Cous Cous

Scrambled Tofu Omelette
Corn Tacos with Pinto Beans
Oat Bran Muffins with Soymilk
Brown Rice with Green Peas and Tofu
Tempeh Burgers on Whole Wheat Bun
Whole Grain Bread with Peanut Butter & Jelly

Noodles with Sesame Seeds
Oatmeal with Sunflower Seeds
Brown Rice with Almonds & Cashews
Avocado, Sprouts & Almond Butter on WW Bread
Corn or Wheat Flakes w/chopped Almonds & Filberts
Chickpea Hummus (made w/Sesame Seed Butter) on Pita

Legumes
Chickpeas
Soy Beans (Tofu)
Lentils   Mungs
Alfalfa Sprouts
Kidney Beans

Tofu Yogurt with Walnuts
Tofu Cutlets with Green Beans Almondine
Sunflower Almond Paté & Sprouts on Pita
Meatless (T.V.P.) Loaf with Tahini Dressing

Nuts & Seeds
Sunflower
Sesame (Tahini)
Nut Butters
Peanuts
Almonds

process vastly increases the availability of the protein and can raise the vitamin content of these valuable foods by several hundred per cent. [120] The digestibility of beans and seeds also improves greatly as the enzymes activated by the sprouting process change the starches to simpler sugars.

Alfalfa and mung bean sprouts can be grown in a jar on the kitchen window sill, or purchased at the supermarket. Serve them as nutritious garnishes to salads and sandwiches.

Sprouting is a fine educational project for children to do themselves. Sprouting teaches kids to value and enjoy the miracle of growing food. Instructions for sprouting grains and legumes, as well as recipe ideas for serving them, are found in most vegetarian cookbooks, health food stores, and are available from the vegetarian societies listed at the end of this book.

Resist the temptation to eat more than three ounces of sprouts daily, as there are plant alkaloids, especially canavanine in alfalfa sprouts, that may cause adverse effects when consumed in excessively large amounts.

From grains to greens, we've examined protein. In my many years of medical practice, I have never seen a case of protein deficiency in a vegetarian. Hopefully, this section has allayed any cases of "protein panic," and has increased your confidence in the nutritional adequacy of the vegan diet.

So now, let's get "down to earth," and consider some "elemental" ideas about - Minerals.

II. MINERALS

Like all animals on this planet, our body cells require metallic elements from the Earth's crust to function properly. Although present in minute quantities, metals like iron, calcium, zinc, selenium, and others, play crucial roles in the chemical reactions of life. Fortunately, these elements are present in the soils in which our food plants are grown. As the plants grow, they take up these minerals and present them to us in the delicious offerings of vegan cuisine.

"The Salt of the Earth" - SODIUM and POTASSIUM

Some vital minerals, like sodium and potassium, are easy to come by, as the vegan diet abounds with them in a far healthier balance than does the meat-based diet. In fact, as was mentioned earlier in this text,

SODIUM and POTASSIUM CONTENTS OF VEGAN vs. ANIMAL FOODS

Foods	Amount (grams)	Potassium (mg.)	Sodium (mg.)
Vegan Foods			
Beans, navy, dry	100	1196	19
Apple	150	152	1
Lettuce, leaf	100	264	9
Oatmeal	28	98	.7
Broccoli	100	382	15
Animal Foods			
Pizza, sausage	100	114	647
Salisbury steak, 3-course frozen dinner, Swanson	45	545	1680
Hamburger, (McDonald's)	102	142	520
Tuna, canned	100	301	800
Cheese, American	14	11	159

the favorable balance of potassium to sodium is especially healthful for the blood pressure, and is probably a main factor in the delightfully low-to-normal blood pressure seen in so many vegans.[121] As mentioned, their low rates of heart attacks and strokes probably reflect the favorable "K Factor" (potassium/sodium ratio) of the vegan diet, as well as the low fat content.

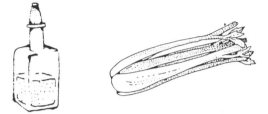

NOTE - Although vegan cuisine is relatively low in sodium, a word of caution is in order about tamari and other soy sauces. These condiments are rich in sodium. One tablespoon of tamari contains an entire day's sodium intake for the average adult. Consequently, tamari and other soy sauces should be used sparingly, especially by those who have problems with their heart, kidneys, blood pressure, or fluid retention. There are some low sodium soy sauce analogs available ("liquid aminos, vegetable bouillon, etc.) - check at the health food store.

CALCIUM, IRON, and ZINC

Calcium, iron, and zinc deserve special mention, as well as the foods that contain them. Remember, the key to adequate mineral intake is realizing that the main mineral sources of the vegan diet are **GREEN and YELLOW VEGETABLES, GRAINS, DRIED FRUITS, and SEA VEGETABLES.** Thus, fresh salads and steamed vegetables should be prepared daily in a balanced vegan diet, with occasional appearances by sea vegetables in salads, and whole grains in cereals, breads, and pastas.

CALCIUM

This vital element, necessary for muscle contraction, blood clotting, and many other vital functions, is amply available in greens, legumes, nuts and seeds.

Although the United States R.D.A. for calcium for adults is 1200 milligrams, this is probably an artifact of the calcium- wasting nature of the high protein, meat-based, American style diet. The World Health Organization, with what many feel is a more appropriate view of human nutrition, recommends a more modest protein intake, 29 grams versus 56, and thus only 500 milligrams of calcium per day. Following the vegan sample meal plans, an average of 800 to 1200 milligrams of calcium is easy to obtain. Numerous medical studies have shown that the intake of calcium on a vegan diet is entirely adequate [122], and that true calcium deficiency on a vegan diet has never been reported.

As presented in "Now How, Brown Cow?," cow's milk is **not** a wholesome and health-promoting source of calcium. Be wise and get your calcium from the same place that the cow gets hers; out of the greens, grains and legumes that grow so beautifully from the earth.

Although concern has been expressed that some forms of calcium may be bound up with plant substances, like phytate and oxalate, and thus are not as readily absorbed, studies by Dr. Lindsay Allen [123] have shown these concerns are not borne out in "real people," eating whole foods. It seems that the human intestine is marvelously adaptable in its range of abilities to absorb calcium. If more calcium is needed by the body, the intestine absorbs more; if excessive calcium is consumed, the intestine absorbs less.

Most people find the natural "packaging" for calcium listed below as more healthful, convenient, and certainly more tasty...

Green leafy vegetables: Collards, kale, (1 cup of either of these greens, cooked, has approximately the same usable calcium as a six-ounce glass of cow's milk, with no troublesome fat or phosphate load). Broccoli, mustard greens, and swiss chard, are also "calcium all-stars".

So are the family of **legumes** - beans of all kinds, chick peas, lentils, green peas, tofu (from soybeans - be sure the tofu is precipitated with calcium; read the label).

Nuts provide calcium to the squirrels and to us! Especially enjoyable are almonds, Brazil nuts, and peanuts, as well as the family of seeds - sunflower, sesame (tahini), pumpkin.

CALCIUM ALL-STARS

FOOD	AMOUNT (grams)	CALCIUM (mgs)
Cow's Milk	100	120
Collards	100 (3 1/2 oz.)	304
Kale	100	249
Oats	120	170
Chickpeas	100	150
Almond/ Raisin Mix	100	290
Tofu (Calcium precipitated))	100	150

These natural food sources, especially if combined with calcium-fortified soy milks, and the substantial amounts of calcium frequently present in drinking water, should supply most everyone's calcium needs.

However, for those who wish to "insure" that they meet the (high) U.S. Recommended Daily Allowance, a teaspoon of calcium gluconate or calcium ascorbate liquid mixed into a gravy, or fruit juice or soymilk, which is then sipped throughout the day, would provide (up to) 500 milligrams of easily-absorbed calcium. (Tablets are less well - absorbed than the liquid.)

Calcium supplements are often mixed with magnesium, which is a good idea for mineral balance. A good mixture of the two elements is 250 to 300 milligrams of magnesium to each 500 milligrams of calcium (see the label).

If calcium supplements are used, be sure they are NOT made from bone meal, or oyster shell. These substances are often contaminated with arsenic, lead, or mercury, that accumulates in the bones and shells of these animals.[124]

Beware of taking excessive calcium if you have a history of forming kidney stones!

IRON

This vital element, necessary for healthy blood, is found in molasses/sorghum, dark green leafy vegetables, whole grains, legumes, wheat germ, beets, barley, artichokes, beans, grains, and dried apricots.

U.S. RECOMMENDED DAILY REQUIREMENT:

Adult Males:	10 mg
Adult Females, reproductive years:	18 mg
Children:	
0 - 6 months:	10 mg.
6 - 12 months:	15 mg.
1 - 3 years:	15 mg.

People with increased needs for iron, and thus possibly in need of supplements, include (1) newborns (breastmilk has little iron), (2) growing children, (3) women with heavy menstrual loss, and (4) pregnant women.

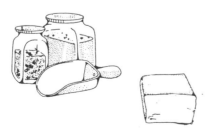

Here are some "iron-clad" friends of the vegan meal planner:

IRON-CONTAINING FOODS		
FOOD	AMOUNT (grams)	IRON (mgs)
Beefsteak	100	3.0
Prune Juice	100 (3 1/2 oz.)	10.5
Raisins	100	4.1
Molasses	15	3.2
Garbanzo beans	100	7.0
Lentils	100	4.2
Millet	25	3.9
Spinanch	100	4.0
Pumpkin seeds	50	3.0
Tofu	100	2.5

Perhaps the simplest way to increase the iron content of cooked foods is to cook soups or gravies in cast iron cookware, two to three times a week. Thus, significant amounts of iron can be simply added to the diet.[125]

The foods listed above should supply adequate amounts of iron for most everyone; but if a finger-stick blood test (a good idea once yearly for children, and several times during pregnancy) shows signs of iron deficiency, more of the iron-rich foods listed should be given, or a supplement providing 15 to 30 milligrams of iron daily should be added, in tablet or liquid form. (Any anemia that does not respond to increased dietary iron, through food or supplements, warrants medical investigation.)

It is well known that **Vitamin C increases the efficiency of the intestine's absorption of iron.** Thus, fresh salads with dark green leafy vegetables (that contain both iron and Vitamin C) and red or green peppers (famed for their Vitamin C content), are especially good "helpers" in obtaining one's iron.

There is abundant iron found every day in the vegan sample meal plans to follow.

ZINC

Zinc is essential to the health of skin, mucus membranes, and the immune system. Fortunately, zinc is found in whole grains, leafy green vegetables, mushrooms, nuts, seeds (especially sesame/tahini), legumes, miso, wheat germ, nutritional yeast, and fortified cereals. A vegan person, eating a balanced diet, should experience no deficiency of zinc. However, if zinc deficiency is suspected through white spots on the fingernails, or slowly healing wounds, 15 to 30 milligrams of elemental zinc can be taken as a supplement.

SELENIUM

This trace element is necessary for normal immune function. It is found in nutritional yeast, broccoli, cabbage, wheat germ, and whole grains.

So remember, fresh green salads, lightly steamed vegetables, grains, and legume products, are the main sources for all the above minerals. Most of these foods are also valued for their rich protein and vitamin content. A balanced vegan diet is centered on these foods, for good reason.

III. VITAMINS

All vitamins necessary for proper cell metabolism and optimal human health, - except B-12 and D (more about them next) - are found in fresh dark green leafy vegetables, and in yellow vegetables, as well as in many fruits.

Enjoying ample amounts of fresh garden salads, raw and steamed green and yellow vegetables, and fresh fruits, holds the key to "vitamin insurance."

At this time, examine the table that follows to build your confidence in the abundance of vitamins in natural, whole foods.

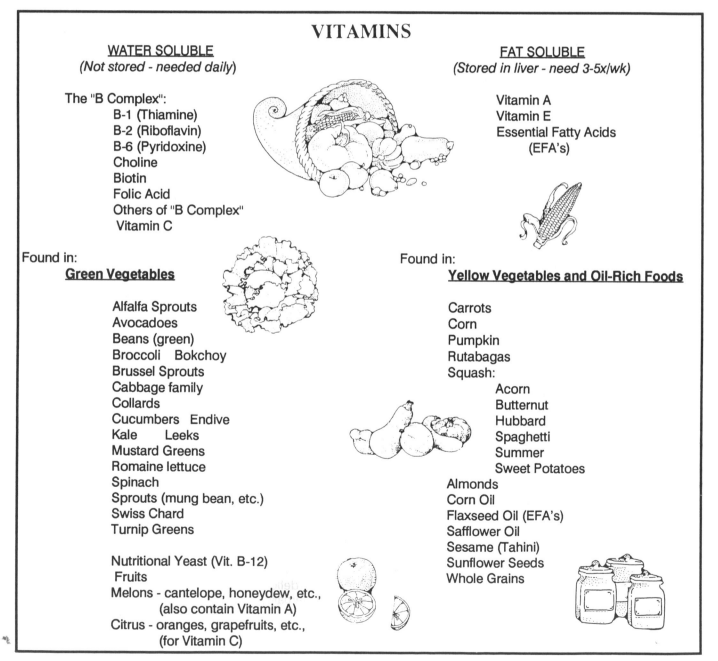

VITAMINS

WATER SOLUBLE
(Not stored - needed daily)

The "B Complex":
  B-1 (Thiamine)
  B-2 (Riboflavin)
  B-6 (Pyridoxine)
  Choline
  Biotin
  Folic Acid
  Others of "B Complex"
  Vitamin C

FAT SOLUBLE
(Stored in liver - need 3-5x/wk)

Vitamin A
Vitamin E
Essential Fatty Acids
  (EFA's)

Found in:
Green Vegetables

  Alfalfa Sprouts
  Avocadoes
  Beans (green)
  Broccoli   Bokchoy
  Brussel Sprouts
  Cabbage family
  Collards
  Cucumbers   Endive
  Kale   Leeks
  Mustard Greens
  Romaine lettuce
  Spinach
  Sprouts (mung bean, etc.)
  Swiss Chard
  Turnip Greens

  Nutritional Yeast (Vit. B-12)
   Fruits
  Melons - cantelope, honeydew, etc.,
        (also contain Vitamin A)
  Citrus - oranges, grapefruits, etc.,
        (for Vitamin C)

Found in:
Yellow Vegetables and Oil-Rich Foods

  Carrots
  Corn
  Pumpkin
  Rutabagas
  Squash:
        Acorn
        Butternut
        Hubbard
        Spaghetti
        Summer
        Sweet Potatoes
  Almonds
  Corn Oil
  Flaxseed Oil (EFA's)
  Safflower Oil
  Sesame (Tahini)
  Sunflower Seeds
  Whole Grains

WHERE THE VITAMINS ARE

For healthy cell metabolism in nerve, muscle and blood, your body needs two "families" of vitamins: those that dissolve in water (water soluble), and those that dissolve in oil (fat soluble).

The inclusion of these fresh fruits and vegetables should greatly reduce, if not eliminate completely, the need for vitamin supplements. If a person wanted to rely solely on the naturally occurring vitamins from the fresh fruits and vegetables in their diet, they could probably do so with little risk. After all, people have been growing up strong and healthy long before vitamin supplements were invented.

Ideally, fresh, inexpensive, locally grown organic produce, cultivated in healthy, fertile soil, would be available to all of us. If one enjoys daily steamed green and yellow vegetables, as well as a generous garden green salad that includes fresh, dark leafy greens, a few carrots, and a strip of dulse (or other sea vegetable) for trace minerals, all vitamin needs (see "B-12" section) should be met adequately and deliciously.

The main rationale for a vegan person to use supplements would be to provide "insurance" if they question the freshness or quality of the produce in their meals. The vitamin content of most vegetables decreases from the moment of harvest, and current commercial vegetable production utilizes long-term storage techniques to permit cross country transport of produce. Thus, a particular lettuce or green pepper may be many days old before it appears on the supermarket shelf, and may be lacking in the needed vitamins.

Most people live in cities, and are thus dependent upon fruits and vegetables with questionable vitamin content. Therefore, judicious use of vitamin supplementation may be appropriate for many people. If one feels vitamin supplementation is indicated, advice and guidance from a physician or skilled nutritionist is advised.

If vitamin supplementation is elected, it is prudent to remember that in the case of vitamins and minerals, as with protein, **more is not better** - excessive amounts of Vitamins A, D, B-6, and Iron, can be toxic. I feel strongly that one should take no more than one multivitamin tablet daily, and, given the "vitamin wealth" of the vegan diet, one tablet, two to three times weekly, should be more than sufficient.

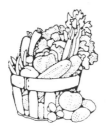

TABLETS, ANYONE?

If vitamin supplementation is deemed necessary, the following preparations appear to meet all vitamin requirements, while being free of animal ingredients:

(The listed recommendations are made on the basis of nutritional adequacy and use of vegan ingredients in their preparations only; the author maintains no personal or financial connections with the listed vitamin producers.)

For Adult Needs:	Solgar* VM 75 Multivitamin. One every 2 to 3 days.
For Pregnant Women:	Bronson* Prenatal One daily.
For Infants:	Solgar "Nutrifort Liquid" One dropper daily.
For Growing Children:	Bronson Chewable Vitamins with Iron and Zinc One tablet daily.

*Solgar products are available at most health food stores in the U.S. - Solgar Co., Inc., 410 Ocean Avenue, Lynbrook, N. Y. 11563.

*Bronson products are available through Bronson Pharmaceuticals, 4526 Rinetti Lane, La Canada, CA 91011-0628.

VITAMIN B-12

Much unnecessary worry has been generated over "getting enough Vitamin B-12." Necessary for development of blood and healthy nerve function, Vitamin B-12 is made (only) by **bacteria**. These bacteria are common soil organisms, and thus B-12 is found on the surface of garden fresh vegetables (washed, but eaten uncooked), in some drinking water, in fermented foods like tempeh, supplemented soy milks, commercial vitamin-fortified "soymeat" analogs, nutritional yeast, and in our own mouths and intestines.[126]

Consequently, clinical problems from dietary B-12 deficiency are extremely rare in vegans. Medical studies by the British hematologist, Dr. Frey Ellis, and Dr. T.A.B. Sanders showed most vegans to have generous levels of Vitamin B-12, even though B-12 tablet supplements were not used.[127]

Most of the concerns over Vitamin B-12 adequacy in the vegan diet seem to be more theoretical than real, and most vegan people seem to grow and function very well without ever taking a Vitamin B-12 supplement.

However, there have been scattered reports of adult vegans with anemia and nerve irritation that did respond to Vitamin B-12. As well, a recent medical study of the nutritional status of vegans[128], showed the serum levels of B-12 of some of the subjects bordered on amounts that could be inadequate in some people.

Fresh garden vegetables, with microscopic soil particles clinging to them that contain Vitamin B-12, as well as foods fermented in porcelain vats, like tempeh and miso, were traditionally rich sources of Vitamin B-12. Now, however, due to industrial production of vegetables, and to sanitation of stainless steel fermenting vats, these food products can no longer be relied upon as adequate B-12 sources. Similarly, nutritional yeast, a food yeast grown upon a B-12 enriched molasses medium, may have great variations in B-12 content from batch to batch, and thus should not be relied upon as the sole Vitamin B-12 source. Nowadays, it pays to enjoy the occasional food which has had active B-12 added to the ingredients.[129]

Therefore, because Vitamin B-12 deficiency, though unlikely, can be serious, and because the measures to prevent it are simple and essentially risk-free, all people using the vegan nutritional approach should assure that they ingest a reliable source of Vitamin B-12 at least three times weekly. This is especially important for pregnant and lactating women, and growing children.

In practical terms, reliable sources of Vitamin B-12 for the vegan consist of:

(1) Vitamin B-12 fortified foods

or

(2) Vitamin B-12 supplements.

Foods fortified with Vitamin B-12, abundant at the supermarket and health food stores, include breakfast cereals, breads, soy "meat" analogs, texturized vegetable protein (TVP), etc. These foods appearing in the vegan diet three times weekly should more than meet all needs for Vitamin B-12.

If Vitamin B-12 supplements are used, oral tablets may be taken, or the sublingual or intranasal gel form are also effective. The daily B-12 dosage should average at least three micrograms, which is slightly more than needed, but provides a safety margin, as not all the vitamin is absorbed into the bloodstream.

The Vitamin B-12 needs of adults should be amply met by the equivalent of one 25-microgram tablet of Vitamin B-12 taken once weekly. Pregnant and breastfeeding women, and growing children, require Vitamin B-12 daily: from .5 micrograms for infants, to 4 micrograms for pregnant women and nursing mothers. For ease of administration to children (and the rest of the family), several tablets can be crushed into a powder, and a small amount added to gravies, soy milk, fruit juices, or smoothies. Of course, the use of standard multivitamin supplement tables would also contain at least 3 micrograms of B-12, and usually more. Be sure to check the vitamin label carefully.

While reading the label, also make sure that the vitamin B-12 is drived from vegetable (bacterial) sources, not from beef liver from the slaughterhouse or from cod-liver oil.

VITAMIN D

Vitamin D is not really a "vitamin" at all, but a **hormone** made within our own bodies by the action of **sunlight** upon substances within our skin. Vitamin D allows us to absorb calcium from the food in our intestines into the bloodstream.

Vitamin D needs can be met with 15 minutes of sunlight exposure on face and arms daily.[130] If this is done, there is really no need to ingest vitamin D in our food. In fact, excessive amounts of this vitamin as a supplement, exceeding 800 I.U. a day, can be toxic.[131]

As you might imagine, people who live in sunny climates usually have little or no risk of Vitamin D deficiency as long as they spend some time outside each day, with sunlight falling on their skin (as opposed to raindrops falling on their heads); fifteen minutes of sun exposure upon the skin is reported to produce adequate Vitamin D supplies.[25] Even in wintertime, a few minutes spent sitting near an open window is a good idea. However, for "vitamin insurance," it may be prudent to add this vitamin to the diet of growing children living in northern latitudes during the winter months.

Four hundred International Units of (plant derived) ergocalciferol (available at the pharmacy or health food store) can be added to soymilk and juices.

The total Vitamin D supplement should be restricted to no more than 800 I.U. daily, with 400 I.U. being quite adequate.

Incidentally, Vitamin D does not occur naturally in cow's milk; it is added at the dairy in the form of cholecalciferol, made from fish oil. Dairy products can actually contribute to excessive doses of this vitamin.

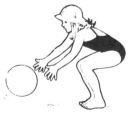

Vegan meals can provide sufficient protein, calcium, and iron. Here is a nutritional analysis of two full days of vegan cuisine. Remember, this is just a suggested pattern. There are endless variations of these themes:

SAMPLE MENU

DAY ONE

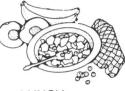

BREAKFAST:

3/4 cup Whole Grain Cereal,
(Rolled Oat Granola, Multi-grain Hot Cereal, etc.)
Topped by Fruit, Chopped Almonds and Raisins,
with 1/2 cup Soy Milk or Sunflower Milk made fresh in the blender;

PROTEIN: 8 g. CALCIUM: 100 mgs. IRON: 2 mgs.

LUNCH:

Medium Green Salad - with fresh Carrots, 1/4 cup Alfalfa Sprouts,
Tahini Dressing and Tofu (4 oz.) Cutlet Sandwich - 2 slices Whole Grain Bread,
"trimmings" of Lettuce, Tomatoes, Soy Mayonnaise.

PROTEIN: 30 g. CALCIUM: 440 mgs. IRON: 10 mgs.

DINNER:

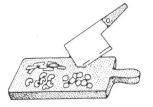

Soup (1 cup) - Bean/Barley/Vegetable, etc.;
Garden Green Salad Italian Dressing;
Vegetable/Grain combination main dish (6 oz. serving)
(with an added legume feature like Tofu,
Lentils, Beans, Sprouts, Chickpeas, etc.);
for example,
Tofu/Millet Loaf w/Carrot, Onion, & Peppers, or
Oriental-Style stir-fried Vegetables
with Tofu and Cashews. Serve over 1 cup Noodles or Rice;
Side dishes of 1 cup steamed Broccoli and/or Carrots with Nutritional Yeast Gravy

PROTEIN: 32 g. CALCIUM: 460 mgs. IRON: 13 mgs.

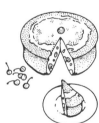

SNACKS:

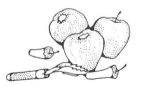

3/4 cup Almond and Raisin mix consumed during the day,
plus any of the following, if desired:
Fruits, Frozen Juice "Pops",
Fruit or Vegetable Juices,
Fruit Smoothies,
Vegan Baked Goods - Apple Pie, Banana Bread, etc.
Popcorn

PROTEIN: 5 g. CALCIUM: 200 mg. IRON: 5 mg.

When thirsty, enjoy liberal amounts of pure water and fruit and vegetable juices.

DAY TWO

BREAKFAST:

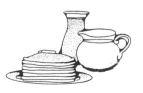

4 Whole Wheat Pancakes (4" diameter) topped with Maple Syrup and/or
Fruit Spread (Apple Butter, Peach Compote, etc.)
4-ounce glass Soy Milk. Fruit Juice,
Coffee substitute (Postum, Cafix, Pero, etc.), or Herbal Tea.

PROTEIN 18 gms. CALCIUM 180 mgs. IRON 2 mgs.

LUNCH:

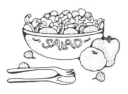

One bowl Tossed Salad with 2 tablespoons Tahini Dressing;
One sandwich (2 slices Whole Wheat, Pumpernickel, Rye Bread,
or Whole Wheat Pita)
with 1/2 cup Hummus (Chick Pea Spread), Lettuce, Tomato, 1/4 cup
Alfalfa Sprouts, Onion:
or 2 tablespoons Peanut Butter with Banana & Raisins
4-oz. glass Soy Milk (Edensoy, Ah Soy, etc.)

PROTEIN : 27 gms. CALCIUM: 400 mgs. IRON: 10 mgs.

DINNER:

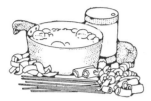

Medium Garden Green Salad with Vinegar/Nutritional Yeast Dressing;
6 oz. Whole Wheat or Artichoke Spaghetti w/Tomato Sauce (with Tofu,
TVP and Mushrooms);
2 slices WholeGrain Bread with Garlic Spread;
or One 8 oz. bowl Red-Bean Chili with 2 slices Whole Grain or Rye Bread and
1 cup Steamed Collards and Yellow Squash,
topped with Tomato Sauce or Mushroom Gravy

PROTEIN: 28 gms. CALCIUM: 420 mgs. IRON: 13 mgs.

SNACKS:

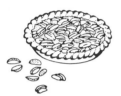

3/4 cup Almond and Raisin Mix and any of the following:
       3 Peanut Butter/Oatmeal Cookies
       4 oz. bowl Oat Granola and Soy Milk
       Vegan Baked Goods
Garden Green Salads

PROTEIN 5 gms. CALCIUM 200 mgs. IRON 5 mgs.

By the end of the day, one would have consumed:

More than 75 grams of (slowly absorbed vegetable) **protein**,

over 900 milligrams of **calcium** and

at least 30 milligrams of **iron**,

all of which meet the Recommended Daily Allowances for adults.

Pregnant women and adolescent children, and others desiring more calcium, can enjoy an additional tofu sandwich, enriched fruit smoothie, slice of whole wheat bread with chick-pea spread (hummus), or peanut butter, or a bowl of cereal with the "Nutrition Booster Topping" (see Appendices).

Anyone on a full, balanced vegan diet should be well nourished!

Now, let's consider a "weighty matter" that will be of great interest to anyone fighting the "battle of the bulge."

JACK SPRATT'S SECRET

There is a great advantage to the vegan style of nutrition because these meals contain no animal fat. They are also rich in fiber and complex carbohydrates, and thus, these foods do not tend to "stick" in your fat stores, which causes obesity.

In other words, most vegans find that they can enjoy ample portions at each meal (with extra helpings!) and still become trim and strong! Virtually all medical studies on vegan people find them to be predictably **lean** [132], and not prone to store fat. They reap the rewards of the nutritional principles that made Jack Spratt, who could eat no fat, such a lean fellow.

Your body's cells prefer to burn carbohydrates as their daily energy stores. The burning of fats is not a very efficient one and fat-burning always creates a burden of fatty acids that must be metabolized and eliminated.

When you feed your body pre-made fats, like those found in the yolks of chicken eggs, the marbling in beef, and the dairy products made with butterfat, it seems to want to keep these fatty potential energy sources "in reserve." The storage depots on most people who eat meat and dairy foods are usually very evident around their waists and necklines. The body also stores fat around vital organs like the heart and kidneys, and at surgery, the true fat "balance book" of the body is quite easy for the surgeon to read. A common post-operative observation is, "He was fatter on the inside than he looked on the outside."

People enjoying vegan nutrition rarely are overweight. As shown in a recent Israeli medical study, comparing weight gain in vegetarians and omnivores, the meat and dairy-consuming people gained more weight, even though the vegetarians consumed more total calories.[133] The difference, of course, is that the vegetarian calories came in the form of "clean-burning" carbohydrates, while the omnivores ate "stickier" animal fats.

As you may deduce from this study, all calories are not created equal. In other words, one thousand calories of broccoli and rice (of complex carbohydrates) simply will not create the fat in one's body as will one thousand fatty calories of bacon, eggs, and cream pie! The plant-derived oils in grains, legumes, nuts, seeds, and cooking oils are easier for the body to burn.

Thus, one of the delights encountered early upon graduating to vegan nutrition is the pleasure of eating ample amounts of delicious food, yet witnessing the melting away of unwanted body fat, and the emergence of a lean, trim, better-functioning body.

Overweight men who change to a vegan diet seem to have an easier time shedding excess weight than do women. The reason probably involves the woman's metabolic need for body fat in order to activate female hormones, like estrogen. Due to her genetic inheritance, the body of a woman on the vegan diet can take a bit longer to reduce its fat stores. Eventually, her body will (really, must) yield to the reality that it is no longer asked to metabolize and store great loads of saturated animal fats.

For vegan people who have trouble shedding those "last few pounds," perseverance and "tincture of time" are ultimately "the cure." One can aid the "fat-burning" forces in the body by:

(1) avoiding excessive amounts of **oily foods,** like nut butters and tahini,

2) minimizing **excessive** loads of fruit sugars, and

(3) taking brisk daily walks or low-impact **aerobic exercises** - swimming, stationary cycling, etc.

(4) Realize cooked foods are "sticker" (contribute to weight gain) than raw foods. Emphasize, salads, sprouts, and uncooked foods.

Eventually, the vegan diet will prevail, and soon more pleasing bodylines will emerge. In my clinical experience, vegan nutrition is the most powerful key to overcoming overweight problems, once and for all.

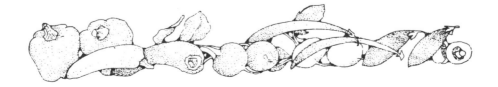

"The average age (longevity) of a meat-eater is 63. I am on the verge of 85 and still work as hard as ever. I have lived quite long enough and I am trying to die; but I simply cannot do it. A single beef-steak would finish me; but I cannot bring myself to swallow it. I am oppressed with a dread of living forever. That is the only disadvantage of vegetarianism."

GEORGE BERNARD SHAW
(1856-1950)

CHAPTER 10

VEGAN INGREDIENTS

A shopping trip to the natural food store to purchase the following "classic" vegan ingredients will help you get started preparing delicious meals. Taking an experienced friend will make the first shopping trip easier and more efficient. You will probably want to have these staple items in your refrigerator or pantry:

BREADS - Breads are excellent sources of protein and fiber, and can be used at almost every meal. "Pocket" pita breads, dark "Essene" breads, whole grain rye bread, "multi-grain" breads, are all popular styles of the vegan "staff of life". However, be sure to eat only **whole grain** bread, avoiding white bread and those containing eggs, milk, whey, honey, or other non-vegan products. Become a reader of labels.

Bread does not have to contain animal products to be light, moist, and delicious! Most bakeries will be glad to oblige a request to prepare a "run" of loaves made with vegan ingredients only - (e.g., whole wheat flour, oil, sorghum or molasses, active yeast, and, sometimes, soy milk) - just give the baker the recipe, such as those found in **THE COOKBOOK FOR PEOPLE WHO LOVE ANIMALS**. Most commercial rye breads are made with vegan ingredients - be sure to read the label on all breads.

Rice cakes and crackers and wafers made from oats, rye, and other grains, are useful bread substitutes for people who may wish to avoid wheat products.

CAROB - A cocoa-like powder (from the locust tree) used in place of chocolate.

FRUITS - Adds sweetness to life (and to food!) Become familiar with the vast range of citrus and other fruits, and begin to use these energy and vitamin treasures for snacks, desserts, and the foundation of fruit-based meals, such as fruit bowls and smoothies.

GRAINS and WHOLE GRAIN PRODUCTS - Brown rice, barley, millet, corn, oats, cous cous, buckwheat groats (kasha), bulghur wheat, and products made from them; i.e., cereals, flour, pastas, breads, etc. Store in dry, covered containers in cool area.

GREEN VEGETABLES - High in protein, vitamins and minerals. Get to know and love them: Collards, broccoli, Brussels sprouts, cabbage, cucumbers, kale, dark lettuce, mustard greens, spinach, swiss chard, endive, zucchini, asparagus, etc.

HERBS - Oregano, basil, dill, sage, rosemary, garlic, ginger, all your favorites that add the spice to life. They work great in vegetable stews, casseroles, and grain loaves.

LEGUMES - Protein bonanzas! Anything that grows in a pod. Of best use to the body when eaten with whole grains; 2 1/2 parts grains to 1 part legumes. Beans of all types (kidney, pinto, navy, lima, soy, aduki, etc), lentils, chick peas (garbanzos), alfalfa and mung bean sprouts, etc. Use in soups, stews, tacos, chili, casseroles, mash into sandwich spreads, etc.

NUTRITIONAL YEAST - Pleasant yellow flakes with a delicious cheesy taste; great on salads, in soups, and sprinkled on casseroles. Contains the entire Vitamin B complex, including variable amounts of Vitamin B-12, high quality protein and trace minerals. A small bowl of nutritional yeast with a serving spoon, placed as a regular fixture on the dinner table, will make Vitamin B-12 supplementation more convenient and delicious for the entire family.

NUTS - High protein "gems" for use in many recipes. Add walnuts to grain dishes, and almonds to vegetable and noodle dishes. Peanuts and cashews are classic additions to Chinese-style stir fried vegetables. Served with grains, nuts markedly increase the protein value of the entree. Of course, nut butters, especially almond, peanut and cashew, and are "nutrient-dense" with oils, protein and calcium, and thus valuable for growing children, and for people who wish to increase their body weight.

OILS - Olive and safflower for table use and baking, coconut for stir-frying, flaxseed as a nutritional supplement. (See "Oils")

PASTAS - A versatile and delicious form of grain goodness. Noodles of all types add substance and character to Chinese and Italian entrees, and are available today in many different flavors and textures. Artichoke spaghetti, spinach-enriched noodles, corn pastas, vegetable "spiral" noodles, broad lasagna noodles, and vermicelli made from rice, beans, and other high protein foods are quick to make and are a convenient "home base" from which to plan a dinner or other entree.

SEA VEGETABLES - Kelp, dulse, nori, kombu, arame, etc., contain Vitamin B-12, iodine, manganese, selenium, calcium, and other minerals. Good on salads and in dressings. Kelp can be used in a shaker to replace salt on the table. Ask where the sea vegetables are grown; avoid contaminated plants harvested from polluted sea water.

SEEDS - High in protein and essential oils. Can be blended with cold water and a dash of sweetener to make a "milk" for pouring over cereal, used in baking, etc. Sunflower, sesame, pumpkin seeds should be purchased raw for eating or cooking, or can be roasted in the oven for toppings and treats. Store in clean, dry, covered containers.

SWEETENERS - Sorghum, maple syrup, barley malt syrup, rice syrup (yinny), natural fruit juices, date sugar, pureed fruits in baked goods, etc. Use them to replace honey or sugar.

SPROUTS - High in protein and vitamins. Easy to make yourself, or to buy fresh at the supermarket. Use alfalfa, lentils, mung beans, sunflower seeds, wheatberries, etc.

TAHINI - Sesame seeds are 35% protein and are a rich source of calcium and phosphorus. Tahini is a "butter" made from ground, unsalted sesame seeds, and is used many places in vegan cuisine; a foundation for salad dressings and sauces, a "binder" for casseroles and burgers, toppings for fruit, and spreads on bread. Often, tahini can be purchased at a reasonable rate, in Armenian or Greek bakeries.

TAMARI - "Classy" soy sauce, made from soybeans, water, wheat and sea salt - aged and fermented. Excellent as a seasoning, but use sparingly, due to its sodium content. Tamari can be found in Oriental food stores.

THICKENERS - Starchy powders like arrowroot, corn starch, oat flour, and agar agar gel give body to gravies, pie fillings and casseroles.

TOFU - High-protein soybean product, sold in four to sixteen- ounce blocks. Rich in calcium; no cholesterol. Extremely versatile, can be substituted for meat, eggs, milk and cheese (see recipes). Can be used to make: scrambled tofu, yogurt, cream cheese, mayonnaise, cream pie, puddings, lasagna, etc.

IMPORTANT NOTE ABOUT PRESERVING TOFU FRESHNESS:

Tofu is sold in most supermarket produce departments, as well as in Oriental food shops. Buy tofu as fresh as possible. Supermarket tofu is usually dated; purchase the package with the date furthest in the future. When the tofu is brought home, immediately open the package, rinse the block, and store in a bowl with fresh water added to completely cover the tofu. Keep tofu fresh by changing the water daily, and using it as soon as possible. Tofu may be frozen, but this reduces the water content and changes the texture, though not the nutrient value. If the tofu has a sour taste, immerse the entire block in boiling water for 10 minutes.

TVP - Texturized Vegetable Protein: Granules made from soybeans; prepared by adding hot water. Adds a hearty texture to spaghetti sauce, chili, soups, casseroles,burgers, etc. TVP is usually fortified with Vitamin B-12.

YELLOW VEGETABLES - High in protein and key vitamins. Have some every day or two in salads, vegetable bakes, steamed in side dishes, soups, etc. Learn to appreciate corn, sweet potatoes, squash (summer, spaghetti, butternut, hubbard, acorn) parsnips, rutabaga, popcorn.

BUYING AND STORING PRODUCE

Buying and enjoying fresh produce to make vitamin-rich garden green salads, fruit smoothies, and steamed vegetable casseroles, should be a delight. The tastes and textures of fresh fruits and vegetables are one of the real pleasures of the vegan diet. Unfortunately, the problem of pesticide residues on vegetables is worrisome for everyone. Various methods for removing pesticide residues have been proposed, such as rinsing the vegetables and fruits in a dilute solution of apple cider vinegar, biodegradable detergent, or fine clay.

The actual effectiveness of these methods is unknown. A more effective maneuver is to peel apples, cucumbers, and other produce before using, as most pesticides are deposited upon the outer surface. Unfortunately, this does result in the loss of the nutrients that are contained in the peels of many fruits and vegetables. Try to make up for it with an extra helping of the peeled fruit or vegetable.

Several companies are trying to develop pesticide solvent/neutralizers for vegetable washing - look for them in the near future.

A desirable solution to overcoming the pesticide problem is to find a source for "organically" grown produce, altogether free of sprays. Of course, growing vegetables in your own own garden is the best possible situation, and many people are using window sills, back yards, and communally owned and operated gardens to create their own organic food supply.

If you are not blessed with a "green thumb," a bit of effort checking the local food growers in your area, will often lead you to a farmer who uses organic methods (their numbers are increasing in response to consumer demand). It is worthwhile to find other consumers with your same concern for quality, unsprayed produce, and then to pool energies to create a "mini-co-op." That is, several families can work together to locate and obtain quality produce, often at lower prices. It may mean a ride out to the country every few weeks to buy fruits and vegetables for yourself and the others when it is your turn in the co-op, but it should be worth the trip.

If you can only shop locally, tell the produce manager of your supermarket or health food store that you want him to stock unsprayed fruits and vegetables, preferably locally grown. Find which produce manager is willing to purchase locally grown organic produce and if necessary, put him in touch with the growers. Be willing to purchase organic produce if your store makes it available. This may mean slightly higher food cost, but, again, food free of contamination is certainly worth the money.

If fresh produce is not available, buy frozen foods rather than canned. The canning process requires cooking the food at high temperatures, which usually decreases vitamin and other nutrient contents. As well, canned foods may contain aluminum or tin leached from the inner surface of the can itself.

When buying frozen foods, make sure they "rattle" in the box. Frozen foods that have thawed and been refrozen clump into one mass. The best frozen foods are fresh fruits and vegetables bought by you in the summer and autumn, and then blanched, bagged, and frozen in your own freezer. For longer and better food storage, keep your home freezer at zero degrees Farenheit (10 degrees below zero is even better).

Food that is **irradiated** to extend it's shelf life may (and usually does) contain harmful "radiodegradation products", like "free radicals", that are dangerous to human health. Irradiated food should be avoided.

For now, let's leave the fruits and vegetables, and discuss a key "family" of vegan staples - grains.

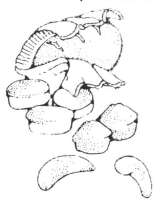

GRAIN IDEAS

In her kitchen, the vegan chef should have large canisters holding many different types of grains. These ancient foods, like rice, oats, barley, millet, and bulghur, should be thought of as ever-ready candidates for the foundation of a fiber and protein-rich main dish.

Here is a brief introduction to the more widely used grains:

Barley	Hulled	A high-protein grain, lightly milled, from which only the outer hull has been removed.
	Pearled	A fully hulled, polished barley that lack many of the nutrients of hulled barley, but cooks in less time.
Buckwheat	Kasha	Related to rhubarb, kasha is the fruit of a plant, not a true grain. Its intense, nutty flavor is a favorite in the Soviet Union.
Corn		A familiar, high-protein seed, the corn plant is actually a grass. The yellow fruit (kernels) are frequently ground into corn meal.
Cous Cous		A processed wheat product, made from parboiled durhum wheat that is milled. High in starch, low in protein, cooks in 2 minutes.
Millet		The "queen of grains," this tiny, round, yellow seed grain cooks to a sweet and chewy texture.
Oats	Rolled	Oat kernels (groats) that have been pressed between huge steel rollers. The "flatness" makes them easier to digest.
	Steel Cut	Oat groats, cut into thin pieces by sharp blades. Frequently used in Scottish oatmeal.
Popcorn		A tough, outer hull surrounding a high water content creates the "pop" of this variety of corn when it is heated. The heat turns the water to steam.
Quinoa		Grain-like seed from South America. Exceptionally high-grade protein. Cooks in 20 minutes. **Rinse very well before cooking.**

Rice	Brown	Rice that has not been bleached or processed is considered "brown rice." Brown rice has all of its original bran and germ, and thus is nutritionally superior to enriched white rice. It also has a chewier, nuttier texture.
	Long Grain	Long grains that cook up dry and fluffy.
	Short Grain	Starchier and stickier, a frequent star in Japanese dishes and dessert recipes.
	Medium Grain	Qualities between long and short grain.
	Wild	Originally found in the Great Lakes area, the seed of this wild, aquatic plant is nutty and delicious, but not a true rice.
Rye	Whole	This hearty grain can be ground into flour to produce pumpernickel and rye breads.
	Rolled	Rye groats (berries) that are flaked or pressed between rollers. Like all rolled grains, they cook faster, and are more digestible.
Triticale		Chewy, high-protein grain - a hybrid cross of wheat with rye.
Wheat	Bran	The outer husk of a kernel of grain, ground off during milling.
	Bulghur	Parboiled, cracked wheat that cooks in 15 minutes.
	Cracked wheat	Wheat berries that are coarsely sliced.
	Flour	Wheat ground between stones.
	Bread	A heavier flour from Hard Red Spring wheat, rich in protein and gluten.
	Pastry	A lighter flour, made from Short Red Winter wheat, richer in starch, and lower in protein.
	Germ	The seed of the grain kernel, rich in oils, vitamins, and minerals.
	Rolled	Commonly seen in hot cereals and granola, wheat berries are flattened by heated rollers.

What a rich selection of nutritious grain products to choose from! So many, in fact, that some people walk into the kitchen, gaze into the pantry, and ponder, **"What do I do with all these grains?"** Here are some useful answers.

First, become familiar with the basic recipe for cooking grains:

(1) Be sure to rinse all grain in cold water several times before cooking. This will remove dirt, small stones, and bitter substances that may coat the surface of the grains.
(2) Use approximately **2 cups water** to **1 cup grain.**
(3) Bring water to boil, add grain, cover and simmer on low heat until water is absorbed.
(4) When grain is done, remove from heat, uncover pot, and allow to cool without stirring.

GRAIN	# Cups Water for 1 Cup Grain	Cooking Time (Minutes)
Barley	3	55
Buckwheat Kasha	2	30
Cous Cous	1	2
Millet	2	25
Quinoa	2	20
Rice	2	40

As you can see, each grain has its own specific cooking time; however, the following variations work equally well with all types of grains (bulghur wheat, barley, oats, rye, etc.), and will add interest and flavor to the different dishes:

a) Add some nuts (walnuts, pecans, a few peanuts, etc.) to the cooking water, and cook the grain with the nuts. Optionally, you can add a few more just before serving.

b) Add some seeds - sunflower, sesame, caraway, pumpkin. You can roast the seeds lightly in the oven before adding them to the cooking water of the grain. Adds an interesting texture and flavor.

c) Cook the grain with vegetables - chop up some onions, corn, celery, chunked squash, or root vegetables like carrots, parsnips, etc.

d) Add some herbs and spices to the cooking water - tamari, miso, Bronner's Vegetable Bouillon, Quick- Sip, or classic spices like sage, basil, oregano.

e) Use combinations of grains - for example, mix rice with barley, millet, rye, bulghur, or oat flakes, etc.

f) Cook the grain with legumes - soak some beans overnight, spill off the soaking water in the morning, and add to the grain before cooking. Grains can be roasted lightly in the oven before cooking for a firmer texture and a "nut-like" flavor.

g) Cook the grains with leftovers, and "freshen" with chopped celery, walnuts, onions, tamari, and cook in a covered pan.

h) Serve with a gravy. Here's some ideas: Use a starch-based body for the gravy; i.e., a little arrowroot, tamari, water, and parsley flakes.

Oat flour, lightly browned in a pan with tamari, water and spices, makes a good gravy base.

Tomato-based sauces and miso-type stocks are vegan classics, as are those based upon tahini or nutritional yeast.

i) Increase the important trace mineral content of the diet. We need more than just a sprinkle of kelp powder on salads and side dishes; learn to cook with "sea vegetables"; i.e., arame, dulse, or kombu (a potato-textured stalk) to rice, soups, or salads.

Though not actually grains, here are a few kind thoughts about their "protein cousins":

BEAN GREAT TO KNOW YA'

a) We should take advantage of the superb nutritional qualities of the entire "legume clan," navy beans, kidney beans, lima beans, aduki beans, pinto beans, as well as peas, lentils, chick peas, and alfalfa sprouts. They are excellent sources of protein, vitamins, and calcium, and their low cost makes the legume/bean family one of the greatest nutritional bargains on earth for human beings.

Add peas to soups, or serve as side dishes - (peas for optimism!); soak lentils and add to salads, combine with vegetables in loaves, or make lentil stew (dal) to serve with rice, vegetables and bread; soak and mash garbanzo beans, add olive oil and seasoning to create "hummus" - delicious spread on bread.

Mash beans into pates and mix them with tamari, miso, onions, or garlic. Serve these on taco shells, pita bread, or crackers.

b) Because they cook much easier when they are soaked in water beforehand, beans soaking overnight in a pot in preparation for tomorrow's soup, chili, or casserole, should be a regular fixture on the kitchen counter.

Overnight soaking of the beans also reduces the problem of intestinal gas experienced by some who consume legumes. Spilling off the soaking water in the morning carries away one of the bean's troublesome sugars, hemicellulose, and thus many people find their bean intolerance disappears.

c) Remember, all legumes can be sprouted! This activates their enzymes, partially dismantling their starches. Sprouting is a highly recommended maneuver that will increase the nutritional value and digestibility of all legumes.

d) Tofu fans will find this versatile soybean product a practical and convenient form of legume protein. It serves as a useful transition food while "kicking" the meat habit, and is a reliable and useful "bachelor's friend."

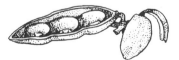

Tofu can be prepared by:

blending with fruit to make tofu "yogurt;"

mashing with tahini, tamari, turmeric, and chopped onions to create tofu "omelettes;"

cubing, marinating, and stir-frying in vegetable sautes;

blending into gravies;

using as a binder in cake batters and casseroles;

mashing and seasoning for a sandwich spread;

slicing and sauteeing as "cutlets";

and in many other delicious and imaginative ways, such as "sour cream" and "cream cheese," that will replace dairy products in the diet.

PUTTING IT ALL TOGETHER

1. Starches (grains, potatoes, pastas, etc.) should be the main calorie (energy) source of your diet, and the center of at least one main meal each day.

2. In planning meals, remember salads and soups add interest and nutrition, and are good vehicles for high-mineral sea vegetables such as kombu, arame, and nori (available at your health food store) and for supplemental Vitamin B-12. Very importantly, find out what foods your family likes the most, (potato salad, pastas, etc.), and make them often. Become comfortable using seasonings and spices to make meals taste delicious.

3. The more you cook food, the greater the loss of its nutrient value. Use foods in as natural a state as possible, avoiding additives, coloring, and excess sugars. Emphasize fresh, raw foods (salads, fruit bowls, sprouts, etc.) over cooked foods.

NOTE - Those who follow the Natural Hygiene philosophy feel that processed and cooked foods are lacking in "vital force," and have no place in the optimal human diet. There may be truth in this impression, as fresh, unprocessed foods are almost always preferable as higher quality sources of nutrition. For children, one can puree or blend fresh fruits or vegetables in the blender or food processor, such as raw apples for applesauce instead of cooked.

In response to proponents of the Natural Hygiene philosophy, although fresh foods may well be always preferable to cooked or processed foods, most people in the process of transitioning away from meat and dairy products are unable or unwilling to move immediately to an all-raw, uncooked diet. Therefore, in this book, cooked and processed foods are included; however, they should be balanced with fresh, live foods, and one's general dietary direction should probably evolve towards enjoying more foods in their uncooked state.

4. Avoid **excessive** amounts of cooking oils and oil- containing foods, such as tahini and peanut butter, and beware of using hydrogenated oils - again, be a reader of labels.

Don't deep fry foods, as it destroys nutrients and increases fat intake to excess. Actually, the less frying in hot oils, the better. Light steamings, **quick** stir-frying in a wok or skillet, or baking, are the gentler ways to serve vegetables.

5. Be aware of what a vitamin and mineral thief water can be. When boiling vegetables, use as little water as possible, and bring the water to a boil before adding the vegetables to minimize the nutrients leaching into the water.

Cooking in covered pans will shorten the cooking time, and decrease the amount of water needed. Of course, steaming, rather than actual boiling of vegetables, is more conservative of vitamins and minerals. This is especially true of green leafy vegetables that lose nutrition through their large surface area. Try cooking vegetables like carrots and celery first, before cutting them up; this minimizes the cut surface area through which nutrients leak out. Save the steaming or cooking water from vegetable preparation to make soup stock and salad dressings.

To minimize Vitamin C loss due to oxidation by air, cut fresh fruits and vegetables just before serving. Because acids will stabilize Vitamin C, adding vinegar to the cole slaw, or tomatoes to fresh-cut zucchini salad, will help preserve the vitamins.

6. Any of the following vegetables can be baked and serve as the centerpiece or side dish for a lunch or dinner meal when baked in a 350 degree oven for approximately 45 minutes until tender: Onions, potatoes, squash, carrots, beets, sweet potatoes, etc.

7. Soups, grainburgers, and casseroles can be prepared in advance and frozen; then defrosted and heated when needed.

8. Simple vegetable sautes are easy to make - start by heating a little vegetable oil (olive, safflower, corn, peanut, etc.) and add fresh garlic and onions. Then stir in the hard vegetables: carrots, celery, cauliflower, broccoli, and finally, the softer ones; peppers, summer squash, cabbage, and mushrooms. Keep frying time to a quick few minutes, and try sauteeing in water with

the slightest coating of oil in the skillet at the beginning. Add some tofu chunks or nuts to the saute and serve over rice or noodles. Side dishes of steamed green and/or yellow vegetables are always a nutritional "plus" to serve with any entree.

WATER

Pure water is essential to good health, and is in ever shorter supply. Have the water in your home analyzed once and then do what you must do - distill it, filter it, or buy it bottled - to be able to trust that it is chemically and bacteriologically safe. Be sure to check for heavy metals, especially lead and cadmium, as well as hydrocarbons from pesticides and industrial pollution.

If you don't have your own trustworthy well or water supply, distilled bottled water or home-distilled water is probably the safest. A high quality, activated charcoal home water filter is acceptable, but be sure to change the filter material often enough to prevent bacterial overgrowth. "Mineral water" or "spring water" may have excessive loads of minerals, depending upon the chemical composition of the rock formation through which the spring flows. Beware of drinking overly large amounts of these these mineral-laden waters.

COOKING OILS

There are health authorities who say that any refined cooking oil is unnatural and detrimental to human health. After all, no other animal squeezes olives or sunflower seeds to extract their oils...

There are some medical studies suggesting that **large amounts** of refined vegetable oils may promote the growth of some cancers. However, these studies, mostly done on animals, involved large amounts of vegetable oil, fed to rats and other creatures with very different metabolisms than humans. One must always be wary of extrapolating such animal studies to "real people" situations.

Also, these studies did not take into account "the vegan factor." This means a person eating in the vegan style eats **NO** animal fats, and thus normally consumes a very low-fat diet, free of cholesterol and many of the saturated fats inherent in animal products. Vegans thus derive **all** their essential fats from the small amounts of plant oils in whole foods. This fact places the vegan person in a different position in respect to vegetable oils...

It is true that the body's needs for essential fats, linoleic and linolenic acids, can be met through eating whole grains, nuts and seeds, and that people can live very well without ever using refined oils. However, I have counseled numerous people with dry, flaky dandruff of the scalp, seborrhea of the face, and dry scaly eczema of the arms and legs - whose skins were saying they were lacking in oil. Within days of adding modest amounts (1 or 2 teaspoons) of olive, safflower or flaxseed oil to the diet, these people's skins responded with a beautiful glow and the disappearance of dryness and inflammation.

Consequently, the modest use of olive and safflower oil for recipes, and minimal amounts of (heat stable) coconut oil for quick frying, is approved. At this time I strongly doubt that a teaspoon of olive oil in the salad dressing will seriously raise the risk of cancer or any other disease **for a healthy vegan who ingests no other (animal) fats**. However, "over-oiling " of any food - with any oil - should be avoided.

One's nutritional beliefs or taste preferences may eventually evolve beyond using oils in the diet, and this is perfectly acceptable. Until that evolution in your food preferences occurs, here are some principles to keep in mind about proper use of oils:

Probably the most healthful oil for general dietary purposes is **olive oil**; it has the best mixture of saturated and unsaturated fats, seems to be gentle with the arteries and helps lower cholesterol levels in the blood. This should be the oil of choice for salad dressings, and low-temperature cooking (stove top sauces, oven casseroles, etc.) With any oil, however, use the smallest amount possible; just brushing the bottom of the pan with a light coating, rather than pouring in a large volume of oil, will leave the food and the palate less greasy. **Safflower** oil and **sunflower** oil are rich in essential fatty acids, and are relatively inexpensive.

An underappreciated member of the healthy "oil elite" club is the light, clear product expressed from the seeds of the flax plant, namely, **flaxseed oil**. Available at your health food store, food grade flaxseed oil contains generous amounts of the essential oils, linolenic and linoleic acid. These necessary vegetable fats are required for a healthy glow to the skin and hair.

Normal nail growth and blood function, suppression of joint and skin inflammation, as well as proper performance of the immune system, also depend upon sufficient amounts of these vital oils. Some investigators have found that many inflammatory conditions of the skin and joints, and even unstable emotional behavior in children, can be benefited by deletion of animal products from the diet and the addition of a small amount (1/3 to 1 tablespoon) of flaxseed oil daily.

For adults with cases of "dandruff", psoriasis, red, swollen joints, and other disorders of dry skin or inflamed membranes [134], one to two teaspoons of food grade flaxseed oil, taken "straight", spread on bread, or mixed in salad dressing, will often improve or cure the condition.

When shopping, remember all vegetable oils decompose in the presence of light, heat, and air.

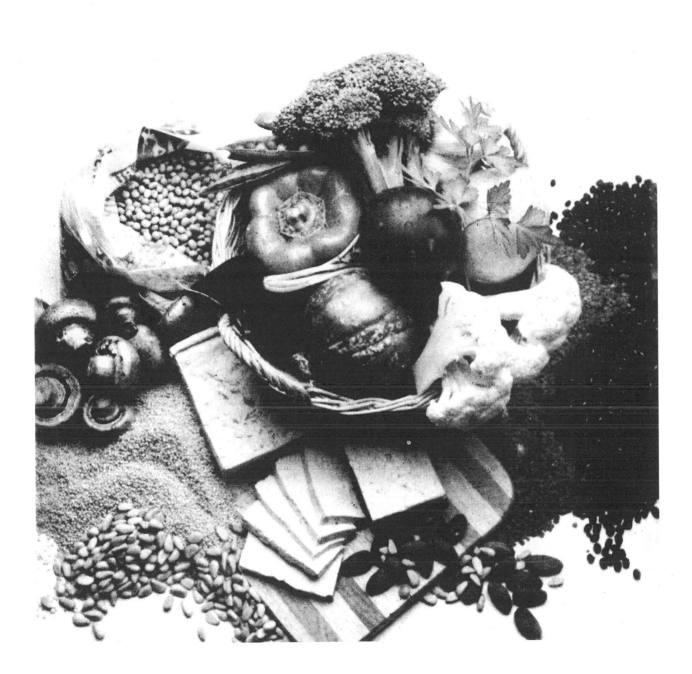

"There is a great deal of truth in the saying that man becomes what he eats."

GANDHI

"The gods created certain kinds of beings to replenish our bodies . . . they are the trees and the plants and the seeds. . ."

PLATO

Therefore, buy and store oil in dark bottles only - never in transparent plastic bottles - and store in a cool place before and after opening. Buy high quality olive, flax- seed, and safflower oils in small enough amounts (250 ml. at a time) so that the oil is used up in a few weeks. A gallon of fine oil is no bargain if you use only a pint in two months and the rest turns rancid.

Do not buy "all purpose vegetable oil," as it is usual- ly pressed cottonseed oil, grown on pesticide-laced cotton plants, and often contains the harmful sub- stance, gossypol. Similarly, "canola oil" is made from rapeseeds, which have erucic acid - not a friendly sub- stance to run through your liver. Neither of these two oils is recommended.

Avoid any oil that has been thickened or processed through "hydrogenation". All margarines have been thickened in this way, and should really be avoided. A slick idea: Rather than spreading your ear of hot corn with hydrogenated-oil margarine (which immediately melts to its liquid state, anyway), why not brush your hot corn or potato with healthier flaxseed or olive oil in- stead?

High temperature cooking with any polyun- saturated vegetable oil, like safflower, sunflower, flaxseed and, less so, olive, denatures the oil, and forms harmful heat degradation products called, "free radicals". These substances can damage vital struc- tures inside your body's cells, [135] and thus, these oils should **not** be used for frying.

The saturated nature of heavier oils, like coconut oil, makes them stable at high temperature, and less likely to form free-radicals. The only role a fully- saturated vegetable oil, like coconut, has in vegan nutrition is, not as a food, but in **teaspoon amounts** at the bottom of a hot wok. Start with a tablespoon of water in the wok, and then add the coconut oil - this keeps the temperature of the wok or skillet lower, as well as the volume of oil used. Many vegetables can be sauteed in water alone, and this is almost always preferred to oil frying.

In conclusion, vegan chefs will find all of their needs for cooking oils met if their refrigerator contains a few, small, opaque bottles of the following four oils - 1) olive, 2) safflower, and 3) coconut. In cases of dry skin, or other signs of oil insuffiency, small (teaspoon) amounts of 4) flaxseed oil can be added to foods just before serving - not before cooking.

OAT BRAN

The beneficial effects of bran upon human diges- tion and general body health has been known for many years. Bran is the fiber-rich, outer covering of whole grains that is not absorbed by our intestines. That is, it stays in the intestinal tube and soon leaves the body. A balanced vegan diet with ample whole grain products contains sufficient fiber to promote normal bowel func- tion, and thus lower the risks of bowel cancer and diverticulosis.

It appears that the fiber of oat bran can soak up more water than the less absorbent bran of wheat. This is an important property...

It is has recently been demonstrated that oat bran, inexpensive and available at the health food store, has especially healthful effects in regulating the fat levels of the blood. Dr. James Anderson, of the University of Kentucky in Lexington, found that eating a bowl of oat- meal and the equivalent of 3 to 6 oat bran muffins during the day, created a dramatic lowering of the blood cholesterol and fat level in patients with artery disease. [136]

As well, a diet rich in oat bran greatly improved the blood sugar control of diabetic patients, many of whom were able to reduce or eliminate their use of insulin and similar medicines. Thus, oatmeal, as well as cookies and muffins made with oat bran, appear to be very beneficial to blood, bowels, sugar balance, and the arteries.

TRANSITION TIME

There is no reason why the change from flesh and dairy products to an all vegan diet cannot be made in a single day. It's as simple as having spaghetti for din- ner tonight instead of the usual meat entree. Your body certainly will not protest against the sudden absence of hormone-laden animal muscle or fat- laced dairy products. In fact, most people who transition to a vegan diet, notice within days feeling lighter, cleaner, healthier, and more balanced.

Occasionally, however, some difficulties do ap- pear during this transition time. Some people feel they experience more intestinal gas, and often blame the legumes in the vegan diet. While there may be an ele- ment of truth to this accusation, the usual cause for increased intestinal gas is more simple.

Analyses show that only 15% of the gas found in the intestine is actually created there by intestinal bac- teria which ferment sugars and starches to methane, carbon dioxide, and hydrogen sulfide gas. Most of the gas in the digestive tract is really **air that was swal- lowed during eating**. You see, in the grain dishes and vegetable entrees, there is air between the grains of rice and leaves of lettuce, and other components of the entrees.

When people eat quickly, and do not chew their food well, they can swallow a great deal of air mixed in with their meals. This process is made worse when large volumes of water or other liquids are gulped down with the meal. Add to this the large amounts of air pumped into the stomach by people who swallow fre-

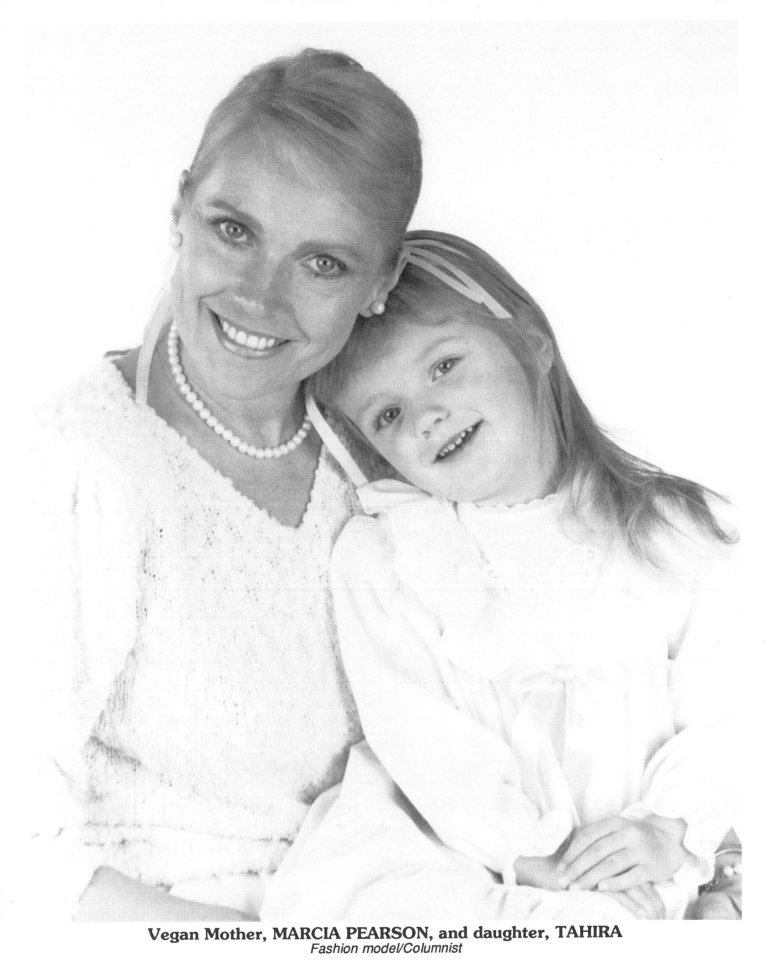

Vegan Mother, MARCIA PEARSON, and daughter, TAHIRA
Fashion model/Columnist

"Veganism is the ultimate personal testimony to non-violence."

quently, like gum chewers, cigarette, cigar, and pipe smokers, and, of course, worried people under stress, and you have the recipe for abdominal distension and discomfort from "gas". All these air-swallowing people can have discomfort or embarrassment from intestinal gas independent of any food in their diet.

The solution to this problem is quite simple. The act of chewing forces air out of the food about to be swallowed. The obvious answer to air swallowing would thus be slow down and **CHEW YOUR FOOD WELL.** As the British say, "Chew your food to a cream", and allow enough time to enjoy the aromas, colors, tastes, and textures of your meal.

Many intestinal and digestive problems, including abdominal cramps and possibly appendicitis, stem from bolting down one's food, with insufficient chewing of fibrous foods. The simple expedient of masticating your food thoroughly, in addition to saving water drinking until 15 to 60 minutes following the meal, will often cure the "intestinal gas" and other digestive problems. (The naturally high fiber content of vegan cuisine virtually guarantees freedom from constipation).

Some distress from intestinal gas can result from an encounter with hemicellulose, a sugar contained in beans. As described, this phenomenon can be greatly alleviated by soaking the beans overnight under water, and then spilling off the soaking water the next day. This washes away most of the hemicellulose that can be transformed by intestinal bacteria into methane and other gases. Keep in mind that, as one stays on the vegan diet, the intestinal bacteria change, and become "used" to the food mixture. Problems with intestinal gas usually become insignificant.

FOOD COMBINING

Some people feel that the combinations in which foods are eaten are important for healthy digestion. Intricate schemes have been devised for "proper food combining," with many interpretations of what the digestive tract really needs for optimal function.

Every individual must determine what, if any, food combinations are best for them. These patterns may vary from person to person, and with each person as time passes, and their body's needs change. Some authors recommend avoiding the eating of protein-rich foods like beans with starchy foods like potatoes, recommending a bean/green salad combination instead - and eating the potatoes separately, at a later time. Others advocate eating only one food at each meal, and some, raw foods instead of cooked foods. Many in the "scientific establishment" declare that food combining is

irrelevant, and that the human digestive system can handle most any food in any order presented to it. All of this means that each person must be a good observer and student of his or her body. If a certain combination of food leaves you bloated and uncomfortable, it is probably an unwise one for you.

DIFFERENT STROKES

Each person must find the meal pattern that makes them feel the best. We should eat according to our body's needs, in response to actual hunger, rather than by the time of day, or our craving for taste sensations. As one becomes familiar with the many enjoyable tastes and textures of "natural" vegan cuisine, especially the desserts and treats, desires for "junk" and other seductive "non-foods" decrease and usually disappear altogether.

Children eating a balanced vegan diet grow up full size and strong. However, children are children, and adults are adults. Although they both have the same **basic** nutritional requirements, there are some important distinctions to be made, dictated by the simple differences in their appetites and size of their stomachs.

It is important that growing children nourished by vegan nutrition be assured of adequate supples of calories, proteins and vitamins. Their meals should accent foods with "high nutrient density", like nut butters, chick pea hummus, pastas, tofu, grain products, fruit spreads, etc., as opposed to "low nutrient density" foods with large proportions of water or non- digestible fiber, like celery and melons.

Fully grown adults, especially those with excessive body fat who need to lose weight, have a different situation. They should accent "low density" foods, like fruits and green vegetables, and avoid oily foods like tahini and nut butters.

For these adults, a frequently successful eating pattern for the day is "fruit-protein-salad." That is, make the morning meal a fruit bowl, or smoothie, with the "protein meal" enjoyed at midday. When these "heavier" foods, like potatoes, grains, breads, and pastas, are eaten in the middle of one's physically active day, hunger is usually assuaged until dinner. The evening meal can then again be light, with fruit or a green salad as the central theme.

Too many people consume a heavy meal at dinner, and then limp loggily to the TV room and then to bed. A walk after eating lunch or dinner is a great idea; it gently increases the abdominal blood flow and the movement of the intestines, both of which greatly aid in digestion.

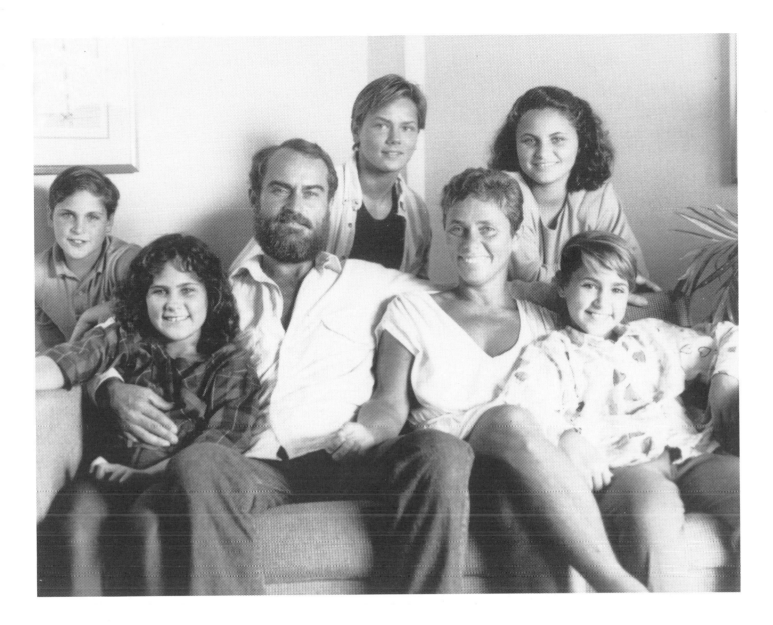

The vegan PHOENIX family

"Veganism encompasses and puts into action all of the love and compassion every peace-seeking person lives for."

John and Arlyn Phoenix have raised their five children as vegans largely for reasons of ethics and compassion. Arlyn explains, "Our family believes in gentleness, kindness, honesty, and truth. That's why our children, River, Rainbow, Leaf, Liberty, and Summer, while having careers in show business, are very careful about the scripts they accept. You can't compromise your soul."

The talented and active children have all been featured in Hollywood films and on television. The family's desire for non-violence in their diets and lifestyles, and the examples they set, have earned then special recognition on the sets where the children perform.

The health advantages of a vegan diet radiate from the Phoenix children. They take no medications or vitamin supplements, have no allergies or serious illnesses, and have never required care by a physician.

"Being a vegan," Arlyn reflects, "Is a wonderful blessing for the whole family. It is a very important step to a higher consciousness. The gift of good health is the 'topping on the cake.'"

A SWEET NOTE

Your "sweet tooth" will not feel deprived as you adopt the vegan style of nutrition. "Chocolate" fudge can be made in the blender or food processor, using carob powder, peanut butter, water, and a sweetener like sorghum or maple syrup. This fudge can be used as cake icing, dessert topping, or frozen for a solid sweet treat. Add carob powder to sunflower milk in the blender for "carob sunny milk" - mmmm!

All vegans who enjoy sweets should know about frozen bananas. Peeling ripe bananas, bagging them in plastic, and freezing them will give you the foundation for many delicious desserts. Chunked frozen bananas, blended into fruit smoothies, increase richness, and when put through a "Champion" juicer, yield a custard-like frozen dessert. For an ice cream substitute, frozen ripe bananas can be served with tahini or fudge topping.

Half a banana on a popsicle stick, or a favorite fruit juice poured into an ice tray, can be frozen as fun treats, and are very simple to make. Freezing a fruit smoothie creates a delicious sherbet.

Non-dairy "yogurt" can be quickly made in the blender with tofu, frozen fruit and fruit juice, and its taste is free of the "sour" quality of dairy yogurt. Tofu yogurt can also be frozen and eaten at a later date. The freezer case at the health food store now has many brands of non-dairy desserts, like Rice Dream and Tofutti, both preferable to milk-based ice creams.

Vegan cuisine offers many baked treats like cookies, cakes, apple pie and banana bread, all made without eggs, sugar, or dairy products.

"HONEY, DON'T"

For general sweetening purposes, AVOID USING HONEY. It carries the risk of botulism, [137] and is a regurgitated insect food, not a human food. Sweeteners like maple syrup, barley malt, and sorghum are far preferable to honey. Fruit juices and fruits themselves can serve as sweeteners in many recipes.

"ON THE ROAD AGAIN..."

(FOOD FOR THE TRAVELING VEGAN)

Any person "on the road" who wishes to eat wisely, safely, and avoid fast food (fat food) restaurants, should travel with a "food satchel" containing the following staple items in plastic containers with **well fitting lids**. Keep these items on hand:

(1.) **Nut and Fruit Mix** - any combination of nuts, seeds, raisins, dried fruit, coconut, etc. Handy in airports, on motor trips, etc.

(2.) **Peanut Butter**

(3.) **Tahini** - mix with water and tamari to make salad dressing, or to spread on bread.

(4.) **Tamari** - use on sandwiches, vegetables, like "soy sauce".

(5.) **Nutritional Yeast** - to mix in salad dressings.

(6.) **Tofu** - store in sealed container under water - use sliced and seasoned, or mashed as a spread for sandwiches.

(7.) **Whole Grain Product**s - pita "pocket" bread,ricecakes, or whole wheat bread, all are conveinient on the road. Sandwich ideas- guacamole(avocado),tofu "eggless" salad,peanut butter and banana or fruit spread, etc.

(8.) **Cereals** - for breakfast - granola, puffed and flaked whole grains, etc. - top with fresh fruit and use soy milk (Edensoy, Ah Soy) bottled nut milks or fruit juice, etc., instead of dairy milk.

(9.) **Fresh Drinking Water**- buy it if necessary, and carry it in an insulated bottle with lots of ice - the ice will melt slowly, and the water will stay cold.

(10.) **Other Beverages** - 100% juice, in small cans or 3 & 6 pack boxes; seltzer or bottled mineral water.

(11.) **Fresh Produce** - if you are on an extended trip, some shopping maybe necessary to replenish perishables, like lettuce,tomato,sprouts, fruits, tofu, etc.

(12.) **Necessary Utensils**- silverware, (including cutting knife, and accessories - masher for tofu and/or avocado), plates, bowls, napkins, cutting tray, and travel drinking cups with lids, straws, plastic bags for trash and compost - and don't forget the twist ties for the plastic bags. For convenience in traveling,keep tahini and tamarin plastic squeeze bottles, and nutritional yeast in a small container with a secure lid.

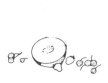
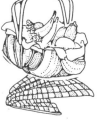

Handy snacks suitable for car, train or plane:

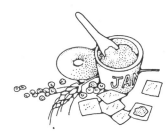

Popcorn
Bran muffins
Unsalted pretzels
Whole grain bread
Whole wheat bagels
Vegan corn muffins
Whole grain crisp breads
Jams and fruit spreads
Fresh fruits and vegetables

When making airline reservations, be sure to specify your preference for a vegan meal. The airlines have become quite familiar with this request, and the quality of vegan meals is definitely improving.

If you find yourself at a restaurant, eat from the salad bar, and look for menu items featuring pastas and side dish selections of vegetables. Order soup, an appetizer, and several side dishes. Inform the waiter that you are interested in meatless entrees, and he may know of a special dish that the chef can prepare for such occasions. Advance notice to restaurant staff is both courteous and effective for vegans dining out. Ask how dishes are prepared to make sure non-animal fat methods are used; i.e., baking, steaming, or broiling. Order sauces on the side.

At the salad bar, choose high-fiber vegetables (broccoli, carrots, kidney beans, spinach, etc.) Beware of cream sauces and other dairy-containing condiments in salad dressings, dessert toppings, as well as high fat condiments; e.g., imitation bacon bits, cheese, etc. When you order a baked potato, avoid butter and keep toppings on the side.

If invited to a friend's house for dinner, give the host as much advance notice as possible of your vegan food preference, and make suggestions for your dinner menu, such as vegetable soup, a large salad, or even a fruit bowl. Most hosts will not feel inconvenienced by a such a request, and the awkward scene of refusing a meat entree can be avoided.

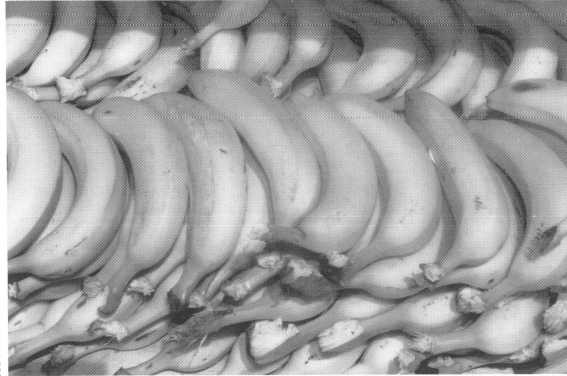

JUDY SUMMERS

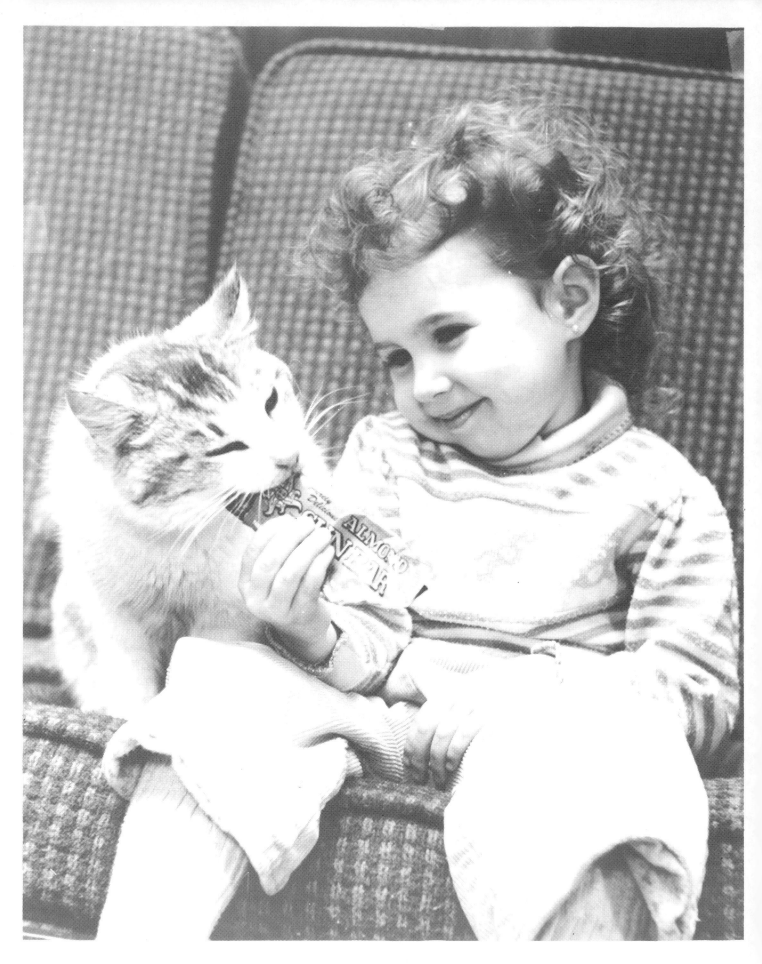

Lifelong vegan, ROSE PEDEN, age 2 3/4, with friend.

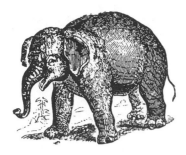
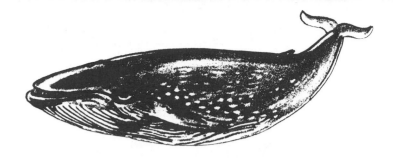
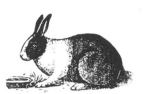
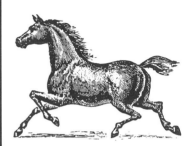

GENTLE STRENGTH

Real health requires more than just the proper foods. A walk in the sunshine every day and abundant laughter are key ingredients; so, too, are enthusiasm about one's work and dreams, the love of friends and family, and joy taken in the natural wonders that Life shares with us each day.

Everything in life makes a difference, just as everything we eat becomes part of us and shapes who we are. Food produced non-violently will make a gentler, healthier world for us and for all the creatures who share our planet.

However, the full scope of the vegan approach of reverence for all life includes far more than food choices. It extends to living gently upon the planet and minimizing the pain and suffering inflicted upon all sentient beings. Thus, many vegan people not only refrain from eating animal flesh and dairy products, but also from using consumer goods derived from the suffering of animals, like leather, wool, silk, fur, tallow soaps, etc.

It is becoming clear that gentleness - toward one's self, towards one's family and neighbors, and to our Mother Earth and all her inhabitants - is essential for true health, as well as for planetary survival. Vegan nutrition, pure and simple, offers itself as the diet for man and womankind to usher in a new age of Peace.

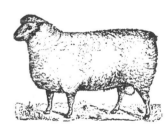
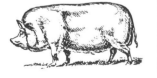
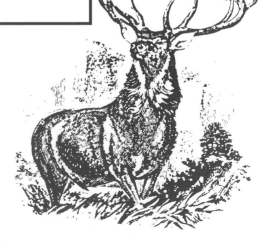
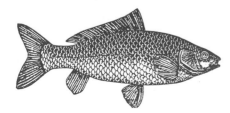
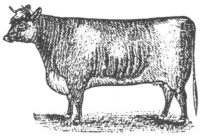
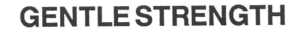

PART 4 - HERE'S HOW

APPENDIX I - DAILY MEAL PLANS FOR VEGAN ADULTS

For certain of these meals, the protein levels may exceed the U.S. RDA, but this is not viewed as a deficit, as the protein is entirely in the form of plant substances, usually bound to complex carbohydrates as in whole grains, legumes, and green vegetables. Thus, the amounts of protein actually absorbed into the bloodstream from the intestines are probably decreased. As well, a specific amount of protein ingested into the body in the form of whole grains, etc., is assimilated slowly, over hours, as opposed to a like amount of concentrated animal protein as in a medium-size piece of steak or fish, that is absorbed into the bloodstream within minutes after eating. It is felt that the sudden increase in blood protein levels following meat ingestion is a greater damaging factor in protein-induced hyper-calciuria and kidney injury, than the total amount of protein that may be ingested during a day of plant-based meals.

In any case, the average protein consumption on a moderate vegan diet is usually far less than that consumed in the standard, meat-based American diet, in which the total protein intake often exceeds 120 grams per day. Thus, among vegan people there is found a lower incidence of protein-induced injury to bones and kidneys. If the reader feels the protein intake from the foods listed in these Appendices are above those desired, the dietary protein presented here can be lowered through omitting servings of high-protein legumes (less than one cup per day), nut butters, etc., and substituting more carbohydrate and oil-containing foods, such as whole grains, avocados, and fresh fruits and vegetables.

Although the total fat content on a given day may exceed the United States R.D.A., it is to be noted that the fats are totally derived from plant oils, and thus are proportionately greater in poly and monounsaturated fats, as opposed to animal products which are notoriously heavy with artery-clogging and obesity-producing saturated fats. Vegan children and adults have far fewer problems with obesity or atherosclerosis.

The iron content of the vegan meals regularly exceed the U.S. RDA. This is of no cause for concern, as a portion of the iron is bound in plant fiber, and thus unavailable for absorption. However, the human intestine, in its exquisite wisdom, seems capable of raising and lowering its absorption capabilities as required by the body, and thus extracting the appropriate amounts of iron. Consequently, iron deficiency anemia is not more common among vegans.

Amounts of calories, protein, iron and Calcium were taken into account, as these are the nutrients most often of concern. The RDA's for all other nutrients; i.e., oil and water-soluble vitamins, potassium, fiber, etc., are met or exceeded by the meal suggestions.

The meal plans are presented with the assumption that a 28-year-old mother, pregnant with her first child, is preparing each dish/meal for herself and her husband, a 32-year-old healthy male, 5'8"tall, 165 pounds. They will both consume the same portions and their nutritional needs will be amply met.

For diet plans and amounts for children, see the author's PREGNANCY. CHILDREN, AND THE VEGAN DIET. The same meals listed here are calculated there for an 11 year old girl and 5 year old boy. However, be assured that a child sharing the "adult" meals given below, in appropriate amounts for their age and using vitamin supplements if necessary, will be fully nourished.

The recipes listed here should provide all essential vitamins and minerals, but a supplement of Vitamin B12 (25 micrograms in divided portions via crushed tablets, drops, etc., during the week) and Vitamin D (Maximum 400 I.U. daily, if sunlight exposure is inadequate) is recommended, especially for children.

Calcium supplements may be used if one attempts to meet the U.S. RDA's, but, as stated above, these foods easily exceed the calcium requirements set by the World Health Organization and should be entirely adequate for anyone employing the "calcium sparing," moderate-protein, vegan style of eating.

The meal ideas that follow are only suggested patterns; there are many variations upon these themes:

MALE, AGE 32 YEARS
Height: 5'8"   Weight: 165 lbs.
Frame - Medium
Active

or

PREGNANT FEMALE, AGE 28 YEARS
Height: 5'5"   Weight: 139 lbs.
Frame - Medium
Moderately Active.

DAY ONE

	FOOD	PORTION
BREAKFAST	Fruit Bowl	6 oz.
	Orange Juice	1 cup
LUNCH	Carrot/Beet/Spinach Juice	6 oz. cup
	Tossed Salad w/Tahini Dressing	1 medium
	Tofu Cutlet Sandwich	4 oz. tofu, 2 slices whole grain bread
DINNER	Carrot Salad	1 cup
	Chinese Vegetable Medley	6 oz.
	Cooked Brown Rice	6 oz.
SNACK	Almond/Raisin/Sunflower-Seed Mix	1 cup

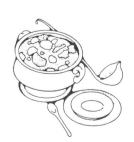

DAY TWO

	FOOD	PORTION
BREAKFAST	Tofu Omelette	4 oz.
	Toast with 2 T. Peanut Butter	1 slice
LUNCH	Mushroom/Barley Soup	6 oz.
	Whole Grain Bread	2 slices
	Tossed Salad	1 medium
	Tahini/Tamari Dressing	1 oz.
	Soy Milk	6 oz. glass
DINNER	Spinach/Mushroom Salad	1 medium
	Chick Pea Loaf	6 oz.
	Carrot/Beet/Spinach Juice	6 oz. glass
SNACK	Aimond/Raisin/Sunflower-Seed Mix	1 cup

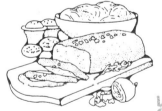

DAY THREE

	FOOD	PORTION
BREAKFAST	Oatmeal	4 oz. bowl
	w/Sunflower Milk	4 oz. over cereal
	Raisins	1/2 cup on cereal
	Slivered Aimonds	1/4 cup on cereal
LUNCH	Carrot Salad	1 cup
	Tofu Eggless Salad	4 oz.
	Rice Cake	1
DINNER	Garden Vegetable Soup w/Barley	6 oz. bowl
	Whole Grain Bread	1 slice
	Broccoli/Tahini Bake	6 oz. serving

DAY FOUR

	FOOD	PORTION
BREAKFAST	Buckwheat Pancakes	2
	Maple Syrup	2 T., on pancakes
	Soy Milk	6 oz. glass
LUNCH	Millet Burger Sandwiches	2 burgers
	Whole Grain Bread	2 slices
	Tahini/Tamari Sauce	1 oz.
	Coleslaw	3 oz.
DINNER	Tomato/Tofu Salad	1 medium
	Potato Kugel	4 oz.
	Carrot/Beet/Spinach Juice	6 oz.
SNACK	Peanut Butter & Banana Open Sandwich	1 slice whole-grain bread, 2 T. peanut butter, 1 banana

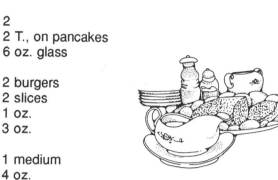

DAY FIVE

	FOOD	PORTION
BREAKFAST	Whole Grain Wheat/Oats Cereal	3 oz.
	Sunny Milk (see Dairy Alternatives) on Cereal	1 cup
	Raisins on Cereal	1/3 cup
	Almonds on Cereal	1/4 cup
	Orange Juice	1 cup
LUNCH	Tossed Salad	1 medium
	Tahini/Tamari Dressing	1 oz.
	Mushroom/Barley Soup	4 oz. bowl
	Whole Grain Bread	1 slice
DINNER	Carrot Salad	1 cup
	Pasta with Beans	6 oz. serving
	Cooked Broccoli	1 spear

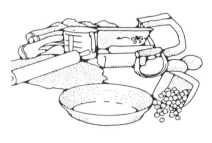

DAY SIX

	FOOD	PORTION
BREAKFAST	Mixed Fruit Bowl	6 oz.
	Orange Juice	1 cup
LUNCH	Spaghetti and Tofu	4 oz. serving
	Carrot, Onion, and Peppers	3 oz. serving
DINNER	Vegetable Loaf	4 oz. portion
	Easy-To-Make Burger Sandwich	2 burgers
	Whole Grain Bread	1 slice
	Carrot/Beet/Spinach Juice	6 oz. glass

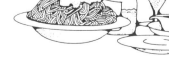

APPENDIX II

DAIRY ALTERNATIVES

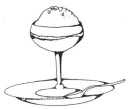

For those ready to make the big "moooove," here's the way to free yourself from the "dairy connection". At breakfast time, when contemplating what to pour upon your cereal, realize it is quick and easy to make your own non-dairy "milks." The secret is to own a good blender, and use **very cold** water in the recipes. With a little practice, a pitcher of sweet, white, frothy "milk," ready for drinking or pouring on fruit or cereal, can be made in five minutes. Try these one morning soon:

For use on your cereal, try this:

Sunny Milk: Start with: 1/2 cup raw sunflower seeds and 1 cup ice cold water. Blend 30-90 seconds until smooth.
Fill blender with cold water, and blend to mix.
Add sweetener to taste.
If sunny milk is prepared the night before, a quick "stir-up" in the blender in the morning will again restore its white, frothy appearance.

Nut Milks: Can be made by adding 1/2 cup nuts; blanched almonds, cashews, etc., or nut butters made of these, instead of sunflower seeds.

Banana Milk: 1/2 blender full of ice cold water.
Slice 2 to 3 ripe bananas.
Add 1 tablespoon of sorghum, barley malt, maple syrup, or other sweetener.
1/2 teaspoon vanilla
Blend well (30 seconds) and pour on cereal.

Soy Milk: 2 cups cold water
8 tablespoons soy powder
Blend with vanilla and sweetener to taste.

OTHER BREAKFAST TIME "MILK BREAKS:"

1. For a change, try pouring apple juice or other fruit juice on your cereal. It's cold and sweet and takes only a little getting used to. This is especially convenient when traveling.

2. Commercial soy milk preparations (Edensoy, Ah Soy, etc., in the refrigerator case at the health food store) are delicious for drinking (ice cold!), on cereals, etc. Liquid and powdered soy milks are available (Soyagen,

Soyamel, etc.), and are fortified with calcium, protein, riboflavin, B-12, and Vitamin D, in levels comparable to those of fortified cow's milk.

(These beverages **must not** be used as "formula" for feeding infants! There are specially constituted soy-based formulas for this purpose).

REPLACEMENTS FOR DAIRY TREATS

TOFU "YOGURT": One 12-ounce cake tofu
(Ice cream substitute) Sliced bananas, 1 frozen, 1 fresh
1 teaspoon sorghum or other sweetener
1/4 cup fruit juice or water

This does not have the sour taste of most dairy yogurts.
Blend at medium speed for 45 seconds until creamy.
Adding strawberries, cherries and other fruits, will create "fruit-flavored" yogurt. Just before serving, add raisins, sunflower seeds, or fruit of your choice (blueberries, diced peaches, cherries, etc.)
Chill in freezer for 30 minutes and serve.

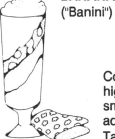

BANANA - TAHINI MALTED: 2 cups water
("Banini") 2 frozen bananas, sliced
1-1/4 tablespoons tahini
1 teaspoon vanilla

Combine all ingredients in blender; blend at high speed for 1 minute, until creamy and smooth. If too thick, add water; if too thin, add more frozen banana.
Tastes like a vanilla thick shake!
Yields 3 cups.

For daily drinks, instead of cow's milk, drink clear liquids like water, fruit juices, herb teas, etc. Without dairy fat in your blood you will become leaner and healthier and help reduce your chances of heart attack, clogged arteries, some cancers, and other serious diseases. The only time we should have milk in our diet is when we are infants, nursing at our mother's breast.

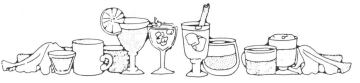

APPENDIX III - RECIPES
The following vegan recipes were created and compiled by Ms. Melinda Patnoi

BREAKFAST

THE BEST BREAKFAST OF ALL:
Fresh fruit (organic when possible) in any form—

from half a cantaloupe, honeydew, or other melon,
to a citrus medley of oranges, grapefruits, and tangerines,
to a bowl full of your favorite mixed fruits

—a light, energy-filled meal to get your day off to a healthy start.

✕ SUN-UP GRANOLA
Yield: 2 cooky sheets

4 cups oats
1 cup cornmeal - fine grain
1 cup sunflower seeds
1 cup sweetener (sorghum, Sucanat,
   maple syrup, raw sugar, etc.)
1/2 cup wheat bran
1/2 cup wheat germ

1/4 cup cold pressed oil (safflower)
1/4 cup fruit juice or water
2 T. vanilla
1 T. cinnamon
1/4 t. nutmeg
1/4 t. salt (preferably sea salt)
1/4 cup water

Variation: Add 1/2 cup sesame seeds or 1/2 cup of shredded coconut.

Preheat oven to 300 F. In a large bowl, combine and mix all ingredients. Place mixture onto 2 lightly oiled cooky sheets, and spread out evenly. Bake for 20 minutes; turn over and bake 20 minutes more. Cool and store in air-tight containers. Serve with non-dairy milks and fruit—or eat dry as a snack.

✕ BRAN MUFFINS
Yield: 1 dozen

11/4 cups whole wheat flour
1 cup wheat bran
1 cup soy milk
1/3 cup applesauce

1/3 to 1/2 cup sweetener
1 t. baking soda
1 t. cinnamon
1 t. vanilla

Preheat oven to 400 F. Combine all dry ingredients in large bowl. Mix all liquid ingredients; add dry ingredients and mix well.

Lightly oil muffin tin by either a light spray of vegetable oil, or lightly brush (using pastry brush) with canola oil; sprinkle with flour. Spoon batter into muffin cups half full. Bake for 25 minutes.

Variation: Add raisins or blueberries, grated apple or grated carrots to batter before baking.

Note about sweeteners: Wherever sorghum is called for, it can be replaced by date sugar, Sucanat, fructose, yinny (rice) syrup, barley malt, or other sweetener of your choice. The amounts of each sweetener used will be approximately equivalent, but the final volumes are to be determined by the taste preferences of the chef.

✕ TOFU OMELETTE
Serves 1 or 2

1 8-ounce cake tofu
3 T. nutritional yeast
1 T. tamari

1/4 t. turmeric
Salt & pepper to taste

Mash tofu in a bowl. Mix in remaining ingredients. Lightly oil skillet using pastry brush. Place batter in skillet on medium heat and press into omelette shape. Brown on one side, then flip over and brown on the other side.

Variation: Add 1 onion, finely diced; and 1/2 sweet red pepper, finely diced
Sauté onion and pepper first. Add to mashed tofu before cooking.

APPLE-STRAWBERRY PANCAKES
Serves 2

1 cup apple juice
1 cup strawberries, chopped
3/4 cup oat flour
1/2 cup whole wheat pastry flour

2 T. soy powder & 4 T. water
  (mixed together)
1 t. baking powder
1 cup strawberry jam

Place apple juice and strawberries in a blender, and blend for about 30 seconds to make purée.

Combine flours and baking powder in medium-sized bowl. Add soy powder mixture and mix well. Add juice purée. Beat until batter is thick and smooth.

Heat a lightly oiled skillet (cast iron or non-stick are best). Pour in 1/4 cup of batter and cook over medium heat until golden brown; then flip pancake over to brown the other side—about 3 minutes per side. Top with jam and fresh fruit.

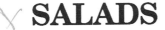 SALADS

CHICK PEA SALAD
Serves 4 to 6

2 cups chick peas
5 cups water

1/8 cup veggie broth
1 onion, diced
1 stalk celery, diced

1/3 cup tamari
1/2 t. garlic powder
1/2 t. cumin powder
1/4 t. oregano
1/4 t. salt

Place chickpeas and water in pressure cooker and cook for 1 1/2 hours.

(Or: Soak chickpeas for 5 hours in enough water to cover, and drain water when ready to cook. Place them in a large pot with 5 cups water, and cook over medium heat for 2 1/2 hours, until soft.)

Drain the chickpeas, reserving the stock for making dressings and soups. Mash chickpeas, and add remaining ingredients and mix well, till creamy. If too dry, add some of the stock. Chill and serve.

AVOCADO MARINADE
Serves 4

2 ripe avocados, peeled and cubed
1 onion, diced
1 tomato, cubed (optional)

Dressing:

1/2 cup water
1/4 cup apple cider vinegar
2 T. creamy mustard
2 T. veggie stock
3 T. nutritional yeast
2 T. tahini
3 T. onion, chopped
2 t. tamari
1 clove garlic, chopped

Place cubed avocado, onion, and tomato in a bowl. Blend all dressing ingredients in blender until creamy smooth. Pour into bowl, chill, and let marinate for 1 hour before serving.

Variation: Add 1 cup of cubed tofu.

CHERRY TOMATO SALAD
Serves 2

1 pint cherry tomatoes, halved
1 t. fresh basil, chopped, or 1/4 t., dried
2 cloves garlic, crushed

1 T. balsamic vinegar
1 t. tamari

Combine all ingredients in a bowl, except cherry tomatoes. Stir well, then gently stir in tomatoes. Refrigerate for 30 minutes to 1 hour. Serve chilled.

TOFU EGGLESS SALAD
Serves 4

2 12-ounce cakes of tofu
2 small onions, diced
2 celery stalks, diced
6 T. nutritional yeast

2 T. tamari
1 T. water
1 t. turmeric
1/2 t. salt

In medium-sized bowl, mash the tofu. Then add remaining ingredients and mix well. Refrigerate to keep cold. Delicious with salad or as a sandwich filling.

RED FLOWER TOFU DIP
Yield: 1 stuffed head cabbage

1 medium head red cabbage
1 lb. firm tofu
1 clove garlic, diced
2 T. nutritional yeast
1 T. veggie broth powder

1 T. fresh parsley, chopped
1 t. dill weed
1 t. onion flakes
1/4 t. salt
Water, as needed

Place tofu in a blender or food processor. Blend until creamy, using as little water as possible. Then add seasonings and blend again. Scoop into a bowl and chill.

Core out most of the inside of red cabbage and set aside. Make sure the cabbage frame holds together. Place cabbage on platter and fill center with tofu dip. When ready to serve, top with parsley. Serve with veggie sticks and/or baked corn chips and/or pretzels. Great for parties.

DRESSINGS AND DIPS

TAHINI DRESSING
Serves 4 to 6

2/3 cup water
1/2 cup tahini
2 T. tamari
1/8 t. garlic powder

1/3 t. paprika
1/8 t. basil
1/8 t. oregano
1/4 small onion, diced

Place all ingredients in blender; blend for 1 minute, until creamy.

TOFU TAHINI DRESSING
Serves 4 to 6

1 cup water
1 8-ounce cake tofu
1/4 cup tahini
1 garlic clove, diced
2 T. tamari

1 T. onion, diced
1 T. lime or lemon juice
1/4 t. caraway seeds
1/4 t. dill weed
1/4 t. garlic powder

Combine all ingredients in blender; blend at high speed for about a minute, until smooth. Add more liquid (water or stock) if needed. Chill and serve.

BLOND MISO DRESSING
Serves 4

1 cup water
1/8 cup apple cider vinegar
2 T. sweetener
2 T. creamy mustard
2 T. blond miso

1 T. nut butter (almond, cashew, walnut, etc.)
1/4 onion, diced
1/4 t. garlic powder
1/4 t. paprika

Combine all ingredients in blender; blend at medium speed for about a minute, until creamy. To make it thinner, add more liquid; to make it thicker, add more nut butter.

MOCK BLUE CHEESE DRESSING
Yield: 3/4 blenderful

8 oz. soft tofu
1/2 cup veggie stock
2 cloves garlic, chopped
2 T. chives, chopped
2 T. mustard
1 T. red vinegar

1 T. nutritional yeast
1 T. tamari
1 T. basil
1 T. oregano
1 T. fructose

Blend all ingredients and chill. Add water (as needed) slowly to blender to thin out dressing.

ITALIAN CREAMY DRESSING
Yield 1-blenderful

8 oz. cake hard tofu
8 oz. cake soft tofu
1/2 cup water or vegetable stock

1 T. garlic, chopped
1 T. red vinegar
1 T. nutritional yeast

Cream all ingredients together in food processor or blender. Chill and serve.

SPICY SAUERKRAUT RELISH
Serves 8

1 lb. sauerkraut
1 green pepper, finely chopped
1 small onion, finely chopped
3 stalks celery, finely chopped

1/2 cup chili sauce, or 1 T. of other hot sauce
1/2 cup sweetener
3 T. lemon juice
1 t. paprika

Mix together all ingredients, and set aside for 1 to 2 hours, then refrigerate. Keeps well.

✕ BREADS

BISCOTTI
Yield: 2 loaves

4 oz. soft tofu
1/2 cup apple juice concentrate
1/2 cup dry sweetener (Sucanat, raw sugar, etc.)
1/8 cup canola oil
1 T. vanilla extract
1 T. almond extract
1/2 cup almonds - ground in food processor into a meal
3 cups whole wheat pastry flour
1 t. baking soda
1 t. baking powder
1/4 t. sea salt

Preheat oven to 375 F. Place tofu, apple juice, sweetener, oil, and extracts in food processor; mix until smooth, using the "S"-shaped blade. Remove mixture from food processor and place in bowl. Then mix together dry ingredients. Slowly fold dry mixture into liquid mixture. Knead into a lightly "tacky-to-the-touch" dough. Form into 2 loaves. Bake at 350 F. for 25 minutes on a lightly-oiled cooky sheet. Then, remove from oven and gently slice each loaf into 3/4" thick slices. Lay slices flat on baking sheet, and bake for 4 minutes on each side. Cool and serve. Great dipping biscuit.

Variation: Roll dough out flat and fill with one of the following filling suggestions:

1. Mixture - chopped raisins, chopped walnuts, cinnamon, sweetener
2. Prune butter or apple butter
3. Mixture - 1/4 cup poppy seeds, 1/8 cup sweetener, 1/2 t. cinnamon

Then roll up, slice into biscuits, and bake.

LIGHT WHOLE WHEAT BREAD
Yield: 2 loaves

4 1/2 cups whole wheat flour
2 1/2 cups lukewarm water
2 cups soy flour
1 1/2 cups whole wheat pastry flour

3 T. applesauce
1 1/2 T. yeast
1 t. sweetener (sorghum, etc.)
1 t. salt

In large bowl, combine water and yeast. Add the sorghum, applesauce and salt. Add 3 cups of whole wheat flour, 1 cup whole wheat pastry flour, and 1 cup soy flour, and blend well. Cover with a cloth and allow to rise for 1 hour.

Add remaining 1 1/2 cups whole wheat flour, 1/2 cup whole wheat pastry flour, and 1 cup soy flour, and mix well. Turn the dough onto a floured board and knead for 10 minutes. Form into 2 loaves. Place in bread pans dusted with dried bread crumbs, flour, or cornmeal to prevent sticking. Allow to rise for 1 to 1 1/2 hours.

Preheat oven to 325 F. Bake the loaves for 50 minutes, switching racks (upper for lower) after 25 minutes.

Variation: Cinnamon filling
1 1/2 cups raisins: soak in water 5 to 10 minutes
1/4 cup sorghum

1/4 cup date sugar
2 t. vanilla
1/4 t. cinnamon

Combine sorghum, date sugar and vanilla in small bowl. Drain the raisins and add to the mixture.

Flatten each of the loaves by hand until it is 1/4" to 1/2" thick. Spread the filling over each flattened loaf, sprinkling cinnamon last. Then, roll up each loaf.

Fold into a horseshoe shape if desired and place in a casserole dish or on a cooky sheet. For crisper crust, brush 1/2 t. oil combined with 1/2 t. sorghum on top of each loaf for the last 5 minutes of baking time, at the same temperature.

(This variation can be used with any whole wheat bread recipe. It is done after kneading the dough, and allowing it to rise. The dough is punched down prior to forming it into loaves.)

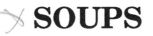 SOUPS

VEGETABLE BROTH or STOCK
Yield: 2 quarts

Make your own stock. Enjoy on cool days as a light soup, or use in recipes where "stock" is indicated:

8 to 10 cups water
2 cups cabbage, chopped
1 medium onion, sliced
4 cloves garlic, chopped
2 celery stalks, chopped
2 carrots, chopped

Seasonings to taste:
Garlic powder
Onion powder
Tamari or salt
Red pepper (optional)
Nutritional yeast (optional)
Kelp and/or other sea vegetables

Bring water to a boil, then add remaining ingredients. Simmer on low heat approximately 30 minutes.

ONION SOUP
Serves 6

8 cups vegetable stock
8 large onions, sliced
2 T. soy powder
1 cup tomato purée or juice
1/3 cup tamari
3 T. fresh parsley, chopped

1 t. salt
1 t. tarragon
1/4 t. garlic powder
1/4 t. basil
1/4 t. oregano

Sauté the onions until tender. Add the stock. Combine the soy powder, tomato purée, and garlic powder; add to the pot. Cook over low heat for 10 minutes; add the seasonings. Reduce heat, cover, and simmer for 20 minutes. If desired, toast whole wheat bread, cut into cubes, and serve in soup; or sprinkle nutritional yeast on top.

GARDEN VEGETABLE SOUP
Serves 6 to 8

10 to 12 cups veggie stock or water
3 garlic cloves, diced
3 large onions, diced
2 celery stalks, diced
2 carrots, diced
3 potatoes, diced (unpeeled)
2 cups green vegetables (Swiss chard, kale, collards, beet greens, etc.)
5 T. tamari

1 cup corn kernels
1/2 cup cooked grain (rice, millet, kasha, etc.)
1/2 t. dill
1/2 t. basil
1/2 t. salt
1/2 t. oregano
1/2 t. garlic powder
1/2 t. parsley

Sauté the garlic, onions, celery, carrots, and potatoes for 4 minutes in a large, lightly oiled soup pot. Cut the green leafy vegetables into bite-size pieces, and add to the mixture. Sauté for approximately 3 minutes, gradually adding the tamari and corn, until the vegetables are soft. Add the stock, grain, and seasonings. Cook for 2 to 3 hours over low heat.

Variation: When soup is done, dilute 5 tablespoons of soy powder in 1 cup of stock; mix into soup to add flavor and thickness.

For a heartier flavor, dilute 3 tablespoons of miso in 1 cup of stock. Add after cooking the soup. Never boil miso, as it loses its flavor.

MISO SOUP
Serves 4 to 6

7 cups vegetable stock
4 garlic cloves, diced
2 large onions, diced
2 carrots, cut into large pieces
2 celery stalks, diced
1 cup small lima beans
2 T. tamari
1/4 t. oregano

1/4 t. garlic powder
1/4 t. salt
1/4 t. parsley
1/8 t. paprika
1 cup whole wheat or spinach noodles (optional)

4 to 6 T. of miso paste

In a lightly-oiled soup pot, sauté garlic, onions, carrots and celery for 7 minutes, until golden brown. Add the stock, beans, and seasonings; cook for 1 to 2 hours on medium-low heat. Add the noodles and cook until tender.

Take 1 cup of stock from the pot; use it to dilute the miso paste, then return it to the pot. Simmer soup for 30 minutes.

SPLIT PEA SOUP
Serves 6 to 8

8 cups water or vegetable stock
2 cups green split peas
1 onion, diced
2 celery stalks, diced
2 large carrots, sliced
1 turnip, diced
1 potato, diced
2 garlic cloves, diced

2 bay leaves
1/3 cup tamari
1/4 cup barley
1 t. sweet basil
1/2 t. garlic powder
1/4 t. sea salt
1/4 t. marjoram
1/8 t. red pepper

Combine the split peas and the water in a large saucepan; place over medium heat and bring to boil. Reduce heat; add the onion, celery, one sliced carrot, turnip, potato, plus tamari and seasonings. Cook for 1 hour, till the peas and all vegetables are soft. Remove the bay leaves.

Transfer mixture to blender, and blend at high speed for 1 minute, until well mixed, and pour into a second large pot. To blend the entire soup will take about 3 to 4 full blenders.

Add 1 clove of diced garlic to one of the blendersful before blending. Add the barley and the remaining carrot; season to taste. Cook over low heat for 2 hours, stirring often.

MUSHROOM BARLEY SOUP
Serves 6 to 8

10 cups water or veggie stock
2 medium onions, diced
2 garlic cloves, diced
2 celery stalks, diced
2 carrots, diced
1 pound fresh mushrooms, chopped

1 cup barley
1/2 cup tamari
1 t. parsley, chopped
1 t. dill
1/2 t. garlic powder
1/2 t. salt

In a lightly-oiled, large soup pot, sauté the onions, garlic, celery, and mushrooms for 4 minutes over medium-high heat. Add seasonings, barley, and the water or stock. Reduce heat and simmer for 2 to 3 hours, adding the carrots approximately 45 minutes before soup is done. To thin soup, add more water or stock.

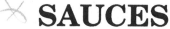 SAUCES

MUSHROOM SAUCE
Yield: 1 quart

1/2 cup flour
3 garlic cloves, diced
3 onions, diced
1 green pepper, diced
1 stalk celery, diced
1/2 pound mushrooms, sliced

3 cups vegetable stock or water
1/4 cup tamari
1 t. parsley
1 t. garlic powder
1/2 t. salt

In a lightly-oiled, medium-sized saucepan, sift in the flour and stir quickly over medium heat until golden brown. Put this aside into a bowl. Using the same saucepan, sauté the garlic, onions, green pepper and celery; sauté for 7 minutes. Add the mushrooms and cook 3 minutes more.

Place the stock and the browned flour into a blender, and blend at medium speed for 30 seconds until homogenized. Add blended mixture to the sauté. Season with tamari, parsley, garlic powder, and salt. Cook on low heat for 10 minutes. For a thicker sauce, add more flour.

NUTRITIONAL YEAST GRAVY
Yield: 2 1/2 cups

1 1/2 cups stock or water
1/2 cup nutritional yeast
1/4 cup tahini
1/8 onion, diced
1 garlic clove, diced

3 T. tamari
1/2 t. garlic powder
1/2 t. basil
1/2 t. oregano
1/2 t. salt

Combine the stock, nutritional yeast and tahini in a blender; blend at medium speed for a minute. Add the remaining ingredients; blend well at high speed. Add more liquid to thin, or tahini to thicken. Season to taste.

Pour gravy into medium-sized saucepan; place over low heat and cook until warmed, stirring constantly.

CREAMY GARLIC SAUCE
Yield: 3 cups

2 T. tahini
1 1/2 cups water
1/3 cup nutritional yeast
2 T. arrowroot powder

3 garlic cloves, minced
3 scallions, diced
1/2 t. garlic powder
1/2 t. celery salt

Combine the tahini and water in a medium-sized saucepan; add the nutritional yeast. Sift the arrowroot powder (through a strainer) and add to the mixture. Add the remaining ingredients, mixing well after each addition. Place pan over low heat, cook for approximately 5 minutes, stirring often, until sauce is thick.

LEMON-MISO SAUCE
Yield: 1 cup

1/4 to 1/2 cup water
1/4 cup lemon juice
2 T. white or mellow miso
2 cloves garlic, crushed
1 t. parsley
1 t. yellow mustard
1 t. olive oil

Combine all ingredients in a small bowl. Chill and serve over salad or steamed greens.

SWEET AND SOUR SAUCE
Yield: 3 1/2 cups

3 cups vegetable stock
(preferably carrot or pumpkin)
3 T. whole wheat flour
1 T. arrowroot powder
1 t. sorghum
3 scallion tops, diced
2 T. tamari
1 t. vinegar
1 t. garlic powder

Toast flour in a lightly-oiled, large saucepan over medium heat for 3 minutes until light brown, stirring constantly to prevent burning. Allow to cool. Add the vegetable stock, sift the arrowroot powder, and then add to the sauce.

Mix in the remaining ingredients, stirring well. Place over low heat and cook for 5 minutes. For a thinner sauce, add a little more stock; to thicken, add a little flour. For creamier sauce, blend at medium speed for 30 seconds.

HOT MISO DRESSING
Yield: 3 cups

2 T. whole wheat flour
2 1/2 cups stock or water
1 small onion, diced
3 scallion tops, diced
4 T. miso paste and 1/2 cup water
1/2 t. garlic powder
1 T. sorghum (optional)

In lightly-oiled, medium-sized saucepan, toast the flour for 3 minutes until golden brown, stirring constantly. Add the stock, onion and scallions, and stir well.

When mixture boils, reduce heat; dilute the miso with the water and add the saucepan. Add the garlic powder and continue stirring until a creamy consistency is reached. For a sweet and spicy taste, add the sorghum.

MAIN DISHES

CHINESE MEDLEY
Serves 6 to 8

5 large onions, chunked
5 garlic cloves, diced
4 stalks celery, chunked
3 peppers, sliced
1/2 head green cabbage, shredded
2 cups mushrooms, sliced
1 cup bean sprouts
1/2 cup veggie stock
1/4 cup tamari
3 T. arrowroot powder
2 T. oil
1 t. prepared mustard
1/2 t. garlic powder
1/4 t. ginger powder
1/8 t. red pepper

In large wok or skillet over high heat, cook onions and garlic in oil for 3 minutes or until onions begin to soften. Add: stock, tamari, mustard, celery, peppers and cabbage. Cook for 5 minutes. Add remaining spices. Sift in arrowroot through a sifter or strainer, and sprinkle into the veggies, stirring constantly.

Cook for 3-5 minutes, till the mixture thickens; then add sliced mushrooms and bean sprouts. Reduce heat, cover, and simmer 3-4 minutes before serving.

Serve over rice or noodles.

74

BOW TIES WITH ROASTED VEGGIES
Serves 6

1 lb. bow ties (pasta)	1/2 cup tomato sauce
1 large red bell pepper, chopped	8 oz. firm tofu, cubed
1 large yellow bell pepper, chopped	1/4 t. salt
1/2 pint cherry tomatoes, halved	1/8 t. pepper
1 medium zucchini, halved lengthwise and sliced	

Heat oven to 450 F. In a large bowl, toss peppers and tomatoes, salt and pepper. Spread on a lightly oiled baking sheet. Roast for 10 minutes. Stir in zucchini and roast for another 10 minutes, or until veggies are tender.

Cook bow ties in large pot of salted boiling water till al dente, approximately 10-12 minutes. Drain.

In a large bowl, toss bow ties and tomato sauce until coated. Add roasted vegetables and tofu, and toss. Season to taste.

TOFU LOAF
Yield: 2 loaves

2 lbs. firm tofu, mashed	1/4 cup tamari
1 cup nutritional yeast, or 1 cup wheat germ	1/4 cup tomato sauce or ketchup
4 slices whole wheat bread	2 T. prepared mustard (not powdered)
4 garlic cloves, diced	1/2 t. garlic powder
2 onions, diced	1/2 t. turmeric
2 carrots, grated	1/4 t. basil
2 stalks celery, diced	1/4 t. oregano
1/4 cup water	

In lightly-oiled, large skillet on medium heat, sauté the garlic, onions, carrots, and celery for 7 minutes. Add 1/4 cup water and seasonings (except mustard, ketchup, and yeast), and simmer for 5 more minutes until veggies are tender. Remove from heat and place in medium bowl. Add mashed tofu to the vegetable mixture, followed by the mustard, ketchup, and nutritional yeast.

Prepare the following mixture:

5 T. nutritional yeast	1/2 t. oil
1 T. tamari	1/2 t. garlic powder

Cut bread into small crouton-sized pieces, coat with above mixture, and brown until crisp. Add to tofu mixture, and season to taste with remaining ingredients. Combine well.

Place batter into a lightly-oiled casserole, and bake at 350 F. for 30 to 40 minutes. Allow to cool. When cool, slide a flat knife along the sides and then turn upside down onto a plate to remove from casserole. Serve with sauce topping or use to make sandwiches.

STUFFED PEPPERS
Serves 10

6 to 10 green peppers, seeded and cored	1 green pepper, diced
3 cups cooked rice, or a combination of	5 T. tamari
1 1/2 cups cooked millet	3 T. tahini or peanut butter
and 1 1/2 cups cooked rice	1/2 t. basil
4 garlic cloves, diced	1/2 t. salt
2 large onions, diced	1/2 t. paprika
1 stalk celery, diced	1/2 t. oregano
2 carrots, diced	Dash of pepper

Preheat oven to 350 F. In a lightly-oiled, large skillet, sauté the garlic, onions, celery, carrots, pepper, tamari and the other seasonings over medium-high heat for 5 minutes, until tender. Add to the cooked grain (leftover baked grain may also be used as a filling). Add the tahini, and season to taste.

Stuff each pepper almost to the top with mix; place them on a baking sheet. Bake for 20 to 30 minutes until the peppers are soft.

Variation: Use the filling to stuff tomatoes and mushrooms instead of peppers.

SIMPLE TOFU CUTLETS
Serves 4

1 lb. firm tofu
2 T. tamari
1/2 t. oil and 1/4 cup water
1 T. mustard

1/2 t. garlic powder
1/2 cup nutritional yeast
Salt & pepper

Drain tofu well of its water. Cut into slices 1/4" thick. Make a liquid mixture of the rest of the ingredients, except the nutritional yeast. Add favorite spices if desired. Place tofu slices into a casserole dish and marinate with liquid mixture for 30 minutes.

Lightly oil a cooky sheet and place marinated tofu slices onto sheet. Sprinkle nutritional yeast on top, then flip over and sprinkle more yeast on other side. Bake at 350 F. for 5-7 minutes on each side; or you can pan fry. Easy, delicious. Variation: Steamed tempeh can be used in place of tofu.

ZITI AND GREENS
Serves 6

1 lb. ziti pasta
1 onion, diced
4 cloves garlic, diced
1 head broccoli, steamed lightly and chunked
1 cup green peas
3 cups tomato sauce

1 cup mixed fresh herbs: basil, oregano, parsley
2 T. nutritional yeast
1/4 t. sea salt
1/4 t. garlic powder
1/4 t. basil
1/8 t. red pepper

Cook ziti in 10-12 cups boiling water for 10-12 minutes until tender, yet firm. Then drain and rinse.

In a lightly-oiled, medium frying pan, stir-fry onions, garlic, broccoli, and peas for about 3 minutes. Then add tomato sauce, fresh herbs, and seasonings. Simmer on low heat for about 5 minutes.

In a large casserole, combine ziti with greens and sauce. Top with nutritional yeast and serve.

EGGPLANT TAHINI BAKE
Serves 6 to 8

4 eggplants, peeled and sliced thin
2 1/2 cups water
1 cup tahini
6 large onions, sliced
3 garlic cloves, diced
1/4 cup tamari

1/2 t. garlic powder
1/4 t. paprika
1/4 t. parsley
1/4 t. basil
1/4 t. oregano

Sauté onions, garlic, 2 T. of tamari, and seasonings (except the paprika) in a lightly-oiled, large skillet over medium-high heat. In a medium-sized bowl, combine the tahini, remaining tamari, and water; mix well, until creamy and not watery. Add more seasonings, if desired. Preheat oven to 350 F.

In two 8x12" baking dishes, pour a thin layer of tahini sauce to prevent sticking; add a layer of eggplant, and a thin layer of sautéed onions. Cover with tahini sauce, and repeat layering. Sprinkle paprika on top of last layer of sauce. Bake for 45 minutes, until eggplant is tender (test with a fork). Delicious served cold in a sandwich.

LINGUINE WITH SWISS CHARD AND GARLIC
Serves 4 to 6

1 lb. linguine pasta
1 large bunch Swiss chard (approximately 1 lb.)
  stalks diced; leaves cut into medium pieces
1/4 cup vegetable stock

4 large garlic cloves, diced
1/4 t. crushed hot red pepper flakes
1/2 cup bread crumbs
1 T. nutritional yeast

Cook linguine in a large pot of boiling salted water until al dente; 10-12 minutes. While pasta is cooking, heat a lightly-oiled skillet and add garlic and crushed red pepper flakes.

Cook, stirring constantly, until garlic is golden (but not brown), about 30 seconds. Stir in Swiss chard. Add salt as desired and 1/4 cup stock, and continue to cook, stirring occasionally till Swiss chard is tender—about 8 minutes. Add additional water if chard becomes dry. Drain linguine. Return to pot, then combine with Swiss chard and toss. Serve sprinkled with bread crumbs and nutritional yeast.

PAD THAI NOODLES
(National dish of Thailand)
Serves 4

8 ounces flat rice stick noodles
1 lb. tofu, firm
1/2 cup green scallions, diced
3 cloves garlic, diced
2 T. ginger, diced

Sauce:

1/2 cup veggie stock
1/2 cup tomato paste or ketchup
2 T. tamari
2 T. raw sugar
2 t. chili or other seasoned sauce
1/2 t. garlic powder
1/2 t. ginger powder
1 cup bean sprouts

1/2 cup scallions, diced
1/4 cup roasted peanuts, chopped
Lime wedges

In enough warm water to cover them, soak the noodles for 15 minutes. Cut the tofu into 1/4" cubes. Combine the ingredients for the sauce and stir well.

Just before serving, place a lightly-oiled, large wok or frying pan over high heat and add garlic, ginger, scallions, and tofu. Stir until fragrant (about 1 minute). Then add sauce, lower heat, and bring to a simmer. Add the noodles (drained) and bean sprouts. Quickly stir-fry noodles until they are soft and well-flavored, and the bean sprouts just begin to wilt - about 2 minutes. Add a little more stock if the mixture looks too dry.

Transfer the Pad Thai to a platter and sprinkle with chopped peanuts and chopped green scallions. Serve at once with lime wedges on the side.

EASY-TO-MAKE BURGERS
Yield: 3 dozen

8 cups of cooked grain
    (options: millet, quinoa, rice, whole wheat
    cous cous, or a combination of these)
3 carrots, diced
3 stalks celery, diced
3 onions, diced
5 garlic cloves, diced
1/2 cup bran
1/4 cup tamari
3 T. peanut butter
3 T. vegetable stock
1 t. oil or 1/4 cup water
1 t. basil
1 t. parsley
1 t. garlic granules
1 t. paprika
1/4 t. salt

In a lightly-oiled skillet, using 1/4 cup water if desired, cook carrots, celery, onions, and garlic, until tender (approximately 8-12 minutes), stirring several times.

Add the seasonings: tamari, basil, parsley, garlic granules, paprika, and salt. Stir in well, and remove from heat.

Preheat oven to 350 F., and lightly oil cooky sheet.

In a large bowl, combine the cooked grain and sautéed vegetables.

Add bran and peanut butter and re-season to taste. Mix well, to reach a consistency that holds together.

Form the mixture into patties, and place them on the cooky sheet. Bake for 15 minutes, turn over and bake for another 15 minutes. Check periodically to prevent burning.

Great served in sandwiches with lettuce, tomato, sprouts, etc.

POLENTA
Yield: 1 loaf

2 cups fine cornmeal
4 cups water
1 t. sea salt

1 t. garlic powder
1 t. onion powder
1/8 t. black pepper

In a large-sized pot bring 4 cups of water to a rolling boil, then turn heat to low, and slowly and gently add 1 cup of cornmeal, stirring all the time with a whisk, spoon, fork, etc.

Add seasoning; then slowly add remaining 1 cup of cornmeal. Stir constantly; you may want to switch to a wooden spoon.

Continue to stir until the cornmeal has absorbed all the water. It should make a very thick, porridge-like batter. If too thick, add more water; but keep it on the thick side. This process should take about 10 minutes.

Then place batter into a loaf dish, press down with fork, let it settle and cool. When ready, you can serve by slicing or chunking, and brown it in a lightly-oiled pan until golden yellow on both sides. Re-season to taste, as desired.

Variation: You can add different vegetables to the batter - mixing well to create a tasty and decorative polenta. For example: green peas, steamed carrots, diced. Sauté garlic and mushrooms. Serve with pesto or a red sauce.

SIDE DISHES

SWEET POTATO PUFFS
Yield: 2 dozen

10 sweet potatoes, peeled and chunked
3 cloves garlic, diced
2 onions, chunked
3 stalks celery, diced

2 cups cooked millet
1/4 cup tamari
1/2 t. onion powder
1/2 t. garlic powder

Place the sweet potatoes in a large pot with 8-10 cups of water and boil for 15 to 20 minutes until soft. Drain the potatoes and mash well.

In lightly-oiled, large skillet, sauté the diced garlic, onions and celery for 7 minutes, until the vegetables are tender. Add seasonings.

Add the cooked millet and seasoned stir-fry to sweet potato mash, and mix well.

Preheat oven to 350 F. Lightly oil a cooky sheet. Drop the sweet potato mixture by the heaping tablespoonful onto the cooky sheet. Bake for 20 minutes.

Variation: Add wheat germ and/or bran (1/2 to 1 cup) to mixture.

CURRIED RAINBOW CAULIFLOWER
Serves 4

1 large head of cauliflower
1 large green pepper, chopped
1 large red pepper, chopped
1 large golden pepper, chopped
1 large onion, diced
3 cloves garlic, diced
1/4 cup water

Seasoning:

2 T. nutritional yeast
1/2 t. garlic powder
1/2 t. onion powder
1/4 t. curry powder
Salt & pepper to taste

In a large pot, one-third filled with water, steam the entire head of cauliflower, greens included. (Keep cauliflower together as a head.) Steam until medium tender; don't overcook. Remove from heat and drain. Place in casserole, flower up.

While the cauliflower is steaming, add 1/4 cup of water to a frying pan, then heat on medium/high. When water starts to steam, add peppers, onion, and garlic. Cook for 5 minutes, then season with remaining ingredients. Cook on low heat for another 5 minutes or until peppers are tender. Remove pepper fry from pan. Then top steamed cauliflower with pepper fry. It makes a beautiful rainbow cauliflower veggie dish.

BAKED BEANS
Serves 4

1 lb. navy pea beans—boiled until tender,
   with a pinch of salt, and drained.
   (Or 1 16-ounce can prepared vegetarian beans,
   drained)
2 large tomatoes, chopped
1 cup tomato paste
1/2 cup veggie stock

1/2 cup sweetener
1 onion, chopped
1 T. chili powder
1 t. paprika
1/2 t. dry mustard
1/2 t. onion powder
1/2 t. garlic powder

Combine all ingredients with the cooked beans; place in casserole and bake at 350 F. for 20 minutes.

POTATO KUGEL
Serves 6

10 potatoes, grated
1 large onion, diced
1/2 cup soy powder
3 T. tamari
1/2 t. garlic powder

1/2 t. paprika
1/2 t. basil
1/2. t. salt
Dash of red pepper

Preheat oven to 350 F. Discard any potato water that has accumulated while grating. In a large bowl, combine potatoes, onion, soy powder, spices. If too moist, add 1/3 cup bran, flour, or more soy powder.

Lightly oil an 8" x 12" casserole dish; put potato mixture into it. Bake for about an hour, checking it periodically, until golden brown on top.

VEGAN CHEESE, ITALIAN STYLE
Yield: Approximately 1 lb.

2 cups water
1 cup rolled oats
4 T. tahini or cashew butter
4 T. arrowroot powder
4 T. nutritional yeast
3 T. lemon juice
1 t. onion granules
1 t. garlic granules
1/2 t. salt

Place all ingredients in a blender or food processor. Blend at medium speed, until creamy smooth; then place in sauce pot and cook on low temperature for 5-10 minutes. Mix will thicken. Cool and chill.

Variation: Add 1 T. mustard for a sharper flavor. Use as a spread or topping; or place in a lightly-oiled mold, chill and slice.

PARSLEY GARLIC POTATOES AND CORN
Serves 6

8 large russet potatoes, peeled and quartered
2 large onions, chunked
1 large can corn kernels, drained
1 cup soy milk or veggie stock

1 cup parsley, chopped
2 cloves garlic
1/4 t. paprika
Salt & pepper

Place the potatoes and onions in a large pot, cover with water, and bring to a boil over high heat. Lower heat to medium and cook for about 20 minutes, or till potatoes are tender, yet firm. Drain well.

In food processor or blender, combine veggie stock or soy milk, garlic, and 1/3 of the cooked potatoes and onions. Pulse until thoroughly mixed, then place remaining potatoes, onions, and corn kernels in a large baking dish.

Top this with the potato purée, parsley, paprika and salt & pepper.
Bake for 20 minutes at 350 F.

DESSERTS and TREATS

CARROT CAKE

4 cups whole wheat flour
2 1/2 cups carrots, grated
2/3 cup apple sauce
1 3/4 to 2 cups sweetener
1 cup thick tahini milk (tahini and water)
2 t. cinnamon

1 1/2 t. baking soda
1/2 t. allspice

1 cup soaked raisins, drained (optional)
1/2 cup chopped nuts (optional)

In a large bowl, combine apple sauce, sweetener, and tahini milk. Stir well. Add grated carrots, raisins and nuts to the liquid mixture.

In a separate bowl, mix flour, baking soda, cinnamon, and allspice. Add dry mixture to liquid slowly, stirring constantly.

Preheat oven to 350 F. Bake 40 to 50 minutes in oiled baking dish.

PINEAPPLE-CRANBERRY UPSIDE-DOWN CAKE
Yield: 1 skilletful

Filling:
1 cup pineapple chunks

Cake:
1 1/2 cups whole wheat pastry flour
6 T. soy powder
   (= egg replacer), mixed with 3/4 cup water
2 t. baking powder
1/2 t. salt

1/2 cup cranberries, fresh or frozen
1/3 cup fruit juice concentrate

3/4 cup fruit juice concentrate
3/4 cup soy milk, seed milk, or rice milk
1/4 cup canola oil
1 T. vanilla

Preheat oven to 350 F. Lightly oil a cast iron skillet. Pour 1/3 cup fruit juice concentrate in skillet. Place over medium heat and bring to a boil. Remove from heat and add cranberries and pineapple. Place in the freezer while preparing cake.

In a medium-sized bowl, sift together flour, baking powder and salt, and then set aside. Blend together egg substitute and 3/4 cup fruit juice concentrate, oil, vanilla, and milk, until creamy. Then fold liquid batter into flour mixture; stir until lumps have dissolved.

Remove skillet from the freezer and pour cake batter over fruit. Place skillet in the center of the oven. Bake 25-35 minutes at 350 F., until the cake shrinks away from the sides of the skillet. Cool cake on a rack for 20-30 minutes.

Invert onto a serving plate. Let cake set a few minutes to absorb all the juices. Serve at room temperature. Do not refrigerate.

RASPBERRY COOKIES
Yield: 5 dozen

1 1/2 cups pitted prunes
1/2 cup water
1/2 cup fruit juice concentrate
1/4 cup hot water
1 T. vanilla

2 3/4 cups whole wheat pastry flour
1 cup maple sugar (or other dry sweetener)
1/4 cup almond meal
1/4 cup all fruit raspberry jam (no sugar added)
1 t. baking soda
1/2 t. sea salt

Preheat oven to 350 F. Lightly oil 2 cooky sheets.

To make prune purée, blend 1/2 cup water with pitted prunes until smooth and creamy. Purée with fruit juice concentrate and vanilla, and add hot water.

Sift together dry ingredients and add to purée, beating just enough to form a ball. Roll dough into tablespoon-sized balls and place on cooky sheets.

Moisten your thumb with water and make a 1/2" impression in the center of each cooky for jam. Spoon raspberry jam evenly into cooky impressions. Bake for 18-20 minutes, until golden. Serve warm or cool.

80

SPICE COOKIES
Yield: 3 dozen

4 cups whole wheat pastry flour
2/3 cup prune whip
 or 2/3 cup apple sauce
1 1/2 cups Sucanat or other dry sweetener
4 T. tahini, mixed with 8 T. water

3 t. vanilla
3 t. cinnamon
1 t. baking soda
1/4 t. allspice
1 cup soaked raisins, drained (optional)

In a large bowl, combine the prune whip or apple sauce, sweetener, tahini/water mixture; add the vanilla and mix well. Stir raisins in.

In a separate bowl, combine the flour, spices, baking soda; also chopped nuts if desired. Mix the dry mixture into the liquid mixture, stirring until it is a smooth consistency. The batter should be fairly dry. Roll batter into small balls, and press down lightly onto an oiled cooky sheet.
Preheat oven to 350 F. Bake 8 to 10 minutes.

LEMON POPPY-SEED COOKIES
Yield: 2 1/2 dozen

1 3/4 cup pastry flour
1/2 t. baking soda
1/4 t. sea salt
4 T. canola oil
 or 4 T. apple sauce
3/4 cup maple syrup (or other sweetener)

1/3 cup pitted prunes, diced
6 T. soy powder mixed with 3/4 cup water
2 T. poppy seeds
1 t. lemon juice
Zest of lemon (grated rind of 1 lemon)

Preheat oven to 350 F. Lightly oil 2 cooky sheets. In medium-sized bowl, sift together flour, baking soda, and sea salt.

In a separate bowl, whisk together oil or applesauce and prunes. Add sweetener, grated lemon rind, lemon juice, and mix well. Stir in poppy seeds. Add wet mixture to sifted dry ingredients and knead until it forms a workable ball of dough. Cover bowl with plastic wrap and refrigerate for 1 hour.

Roll out dough on a lightly floured surface to about a 1/4" thickness. (Do not overwork dough.) Using a cooky cutter, cut cookies and transfer to cooky sheets. Bake for 12-15 minutes, or till browned.
Serve warm or cool.

PAPAYA PIE

Crust:
1 cup almonds (Soak in water 6-12 hours,
 drain liquid, and rinse.)
1/4 cup pecans

1/8 t. cinnamon
1/8 t. nutmeg

Place crust ingredients in food processor, using "S" blade, and grind until smooth. Form into a pie crust in a pie plate, and bake at 350 F. for 20 minutes.

Filling:
3 papayas (small, Hawaiian size),
 peeled and sliced
1 cup strawberries

3/4 cup dates
3/4 t. cinnamon
Pinch of nutmeg

Blend in food processor the strawberries, dates, cinnamon and nutmeg. Add a small amount of water if needed, until creamy smooth. Then arrange papaya slices onto the baked pie crust.

Top with strawberry spread, then another layer of papaya and another layer of strawberry spread. Chill and serve.

Variation: Substitute mango for papaya, and/or: substitute blueberries for strawberries.

FROZEN BANANAS

Peel ripe bananas; freeze in plastic bags. Slice each frozen banana thin, serve with nut or fruit topping.
If desired, roll whole frozen banana in peanut butter or carob syrup, coating thoroughly; then in granola or crushed nuts, and return to freezer.

JUICES AND SMOOTHIES

PINK PASSION POTION
Yield: 1 blenderful

4 apples, cored and peeled
4 cups seedless red grapes
1/2 cup apple juice
1/2 cup cranberries, fresh or frozen
Juice of 1 lemon

Cut apples into wedges. Place apples, red grapes and cranberries in a juicer and extract juice. Then blend all juices and remaining ingredients until frothy.

Pour into glasses and serve. Garnish with a sprig of mint.

BERRY SMOOTHIE
Yield: 1 blenderful

1 cup apple juice
1 cup strawberries, fresh or frozen
1 banana - fresh or frozen
1/2 cup blueberries
6 ice cubes
1/2 t. vanilla

Pour apple juice into blender. Add remaining ingredients and blend until smooth. Pour into glasses, garnish with a strawberry, and serve.

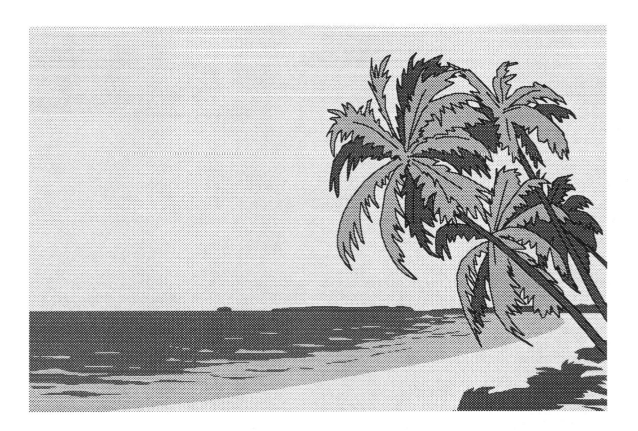

RECIPE LIST

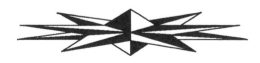

RECIPE INDEX

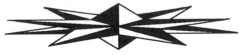

NOTES:

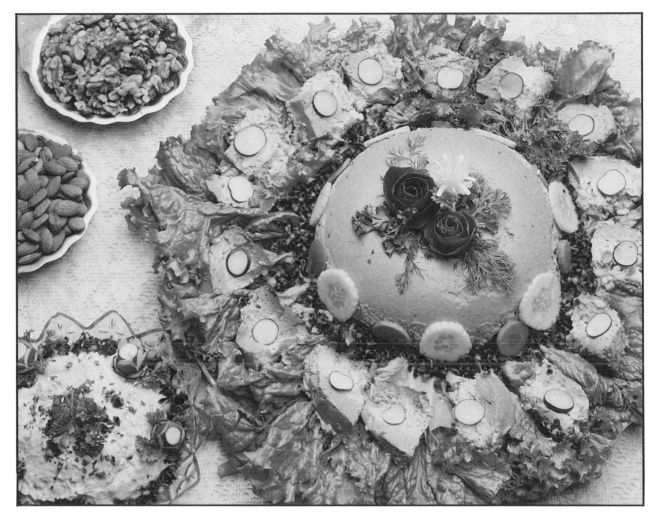

DEAN PAPPAS

"The doctor of the future will give no medicine, but instead will interest his patients in the care of the human frame, in diet, and in the cause and prevention of disease."

THOMAS EDISON

ACKNOWLEDGMENTS

The author gratefully acknowledges the valuable suggestions made by friends and colleagues in the "vegetarian nutritional network" in the production of this work:

Nutrition professionals John McDougall, M.D., St. Helena, California; Agatha Thrash, M.D., Seale, Alabama; George Eisman, R.D., Burdette, New York; Neal Barnard, M.D., Washington, DC; Sue Havala, R.D., Charlotte, North Carolina; and Steven Tiger, P.A., Fort Bragg, California; provided guidance in sections on vitamins, protein, and other vital nutrients. The reflections on calcium contents of foods by Bob Leroy, R.D. (New York) were especially appreciated, as was Keith Akers' inspiring *Vegetarian Sourcebook.*

Special gratitude to Light and Sun, and the pioneering members of Gentle World, Inc., the vegan educational organization, based in Maui, Hawaii, who have provided so much knowledge and insight about the vegan diet and lifestyle.

Recognition is given to the many years of leadership and encouragement of Jay and Freya Dinshah of the American Vegan Society.

Inspiration was, and continues to be drawn from those who work for a gentler world by calling to our attention the treatment of non-human animals—dedicated and caring people such as:

Alex Hershaft, Ph.D., Syndee Brinkman, Tom Regan, Ph.D., Cleveland Amory, Ingrid Newkirk, Melinda Marks, Alex Pacheco, Eliot Katz, D.V.M., Charles Stahler, Debra Wasserman, Chas Chiodo, the Phoenix family, Brian Graff, Mitch Darer, Gene Burke, Linda Levine, Janie Greenspun, Coby and Hans Siegenthaler, Phil Becker, Ruth Maier, Shelly Schleuter, Sherry Schleuter, Barbara Peden, James Peden, Don Barnes, George Cave, Ph.D., Bernie Unti, Doug Moss, Wayne Pacelle, Kim Bartlett and the staff of the *Animals' Agenda,* Gil Michaels and the staff of the *Animals' Voice,* Paul Obis and the staff of *Vegetarian Times,* Holly Jensen, R.N., John and Noah Simcox, Cole McFarland and the staff of *Compassion for Animals,* Bob Barker, Earl Holliman and *Actors and Others for Animals,* Gretchen Wyler, Peter Burwash, the late Cesar Chavez, Deo and Ocean Robbins, Jane Bass, Joanna Macy, Mark Matthew Braunstein, the Baral family, Ellen Sue Spivak, Joel Friedman, M.D., the late Scott Nearing and Helen Nearing, Steve Kretzmann, Frances Moore Lappé, Victoria Moran,

Fred Rogers, Leonard Smith, M.D., the Colluras, Debbie Weidel, Sandra Behm and *PRISM,* Tony Shale, the staff of *The Vegan* (U.K.), Juliet Gellatley and *VIVA!* (U.K.), Judy Summers, Stas, Susan and Les Stewart, D.D.S., Chris DeRose, Jack Carrone, Dinah Carrone, Marcia Pearson and family, Katherine Kinsolving, Walter and Nan Simpson, Tomi Gatling, Lorene Cox, Patricia Lambert, Clive Thomas, Jay Wagner, Michael Fox, D.V.M., Gary Francione, J.D., Winston Miller, Henry Spira, Bill Shurtleff and Akiko, Harry Bromley, Jacques Cousteau, and the many others who care for and love all who live.

Recognition for their inspiring work on behalf of planetary peace and sanity is expressed to Casey Kasem, and to John Robbins of *EarthSave International,* author of *Diet for a New America.*

Extra special thanks goes to two remarkable people:

J. Miriam Greenbaum, for her superb skills, positive attitude, and countless hours at the word processor,

and

Cynthia Lee Pararo, for her imaginative editing suggestions and tireless efforts.

Without their labor and insightful contributions,

VEGAN NUTRITION: PURE AND SIMPLE

would not have been more than lecture notes.

...and appreciation is expressed for the beautiful and magical animals everywhere on our planet Earth, for their reminder of our potential, and of our responsibility...

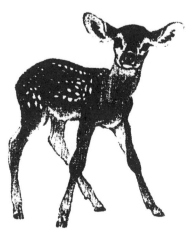

REFERENCES

(1) a. Lappe, F.R., <u>Diet for a Small Planet</u>, Ballantine, Inc., New York, NY., 1976.

b. Journal of the American Dietetic Association, 77: 61-69, 1980.

(2) Hur, Robin, <u>Food Reform: Our Desperate Need</u>, Heidelberg Publishers, 1975, page 95.

(3) a. Tannenbaum, A. "The genesis and growth of tumors. III. Effects of a high-fat diet." Cancer Research, 2:468, 1942.

b. Page, L., and Friend, B. "The changing United States diet." Bioscience, 28:192, 1978.

c. Enos, W., "Pathogenesis of Coronary Disease in American Soldiers Killed in Korea," Journal of the American Medical Association, 158:912, 1955.

(4) a. Hindhede, M., "The Effect of Food Restrictions During War on Mortality in Copenhagen," Journal of the American Medical Association, 74 (6):381,1920.

b. Malmros, H. "The Relation of Nutrition to Health," Acta Medica Scandinavia, Supplement No. 246, 1950.

c. Fisher, Irving, "The Influence of Flesh Eating on Endurance," Yale Medical Journal, 13(5):205-21, 1907.

(5) Akers, Keith, <u>A Vegetarian Sourcebook</u>, G. Putnam & Sons, NY, NY., P. 21-50.

(6) a. Thorogood, M., et al. "Plasma lipids and lipoprotein cholesterol concentrations in people with different diets in Britain." British Medical Journal (Clin.Res.) 1987 Aug.8. 295(6594). P.351-3.

b. Fisher, M., et al. "The effect of vegetarian diets on plasma lipid and platelet levels." Archives of Internal Medicine, 1986 Jun. 146(6). P. 1193-7.

(7) a. Phillips, R., "Coronary Heart Disease Mortality Among Seventh Day Adventists with Differing Dietary Habits,", Abstract American Public Health Association Meeting, Chicago, Nov. 16-20, 1975.

b. Sacks, F., "Plasma Lipids and Lipoproteins in Vegetarians and Controls," New England Journal of Medicine, 292:1148, 1975.

(8) a. Johnson, N., et al, "Effect of Level of Protein Intake on Urinary and Fecal Calcium and Calcium Retention..." Journal of Nutrition, 100:1425, 1970.

b. Allen, L., et al, "Protein-Induced Hypercalcuria: A Longer-Term Study," American Journal of Clinical Nutrition, 32:741, 1979.

(9) Brenner, B., "Dietary Protein Intake and the Progressive Nature of Kidney Disease...," New England Journal of Medicine, 307:652, 1982.

(10) Moore, M.D., Richard, et al, <u>The K Factor</u>, McMillan Publishing, P. 41-119.

(11) McDougall, M.D., John, <u>McDougall's Medicine: A Challenging Second Opinion</u>, New Century Press, P. 202-208., 1986.

(12) Friedman, M., "Serum Lipids and Conjunctival Circulation After Fat Ingestion...," Circulation, 29:874, 1984.

(13) a. Armstrong, B., "Diet and Reproductive Hormones, A Study of Vegetarian and Non-Vegetarian Postmenopausal Women," Journal of the National Cancer Institute, 67:761, 1981.

b. Carroll, K., "Dietary Fat in Relation to Tumour Genesis," Progress in Biochemical Pharmacology, 10:308, 1975.

(14)   N. Tuna and H.K. Mangold, "Fatty Acids of the Atheromatous Plaque," in, <u>Evolution of Atherosclerotic Plaque,</u> ed. R.J. Jones (Chicago: University of Chicago Press, 1963.)

(15)   Values calculated on the Nutrition Wizard, Center for Science in the Public Interest, 1501 Sixteenth St., NW, Washington, DC 20036.

(16)   a   Shekelle, R., "Diet, Serum Cholesterol and Death From Coronary Heart Disease," New England Journal of Medicine, 364-65. 1981.
        b. O'Brien, B., "Human Plasma Lipid Responses to Red Meat, Poultry, Fish and Eggs," American Journal or Clinical Nutrition, 33-2573, 1980.
        c. Weisburger, J. "Nutrition and Cancer - On the Mechanisms Bearing on Causes of Cancer of the Colon, Breast, Prostate, and Stomach." Bulletin of the New York Academy of Medicine, 56:673, 1980.

(16a)   "Circulating Immune Complexes in Infants Fed on Cow's Milk." Nature 272:632, April 13, 1978.

(17)   Taik Lee, Kyu, "Geographic Studies of Atherosclerosis: The Effect of a Strict Vegetarian Diet..." Archives of Environmental Health, 4:14, 1962.

(18)   Shinwell, E.D., et al. Totally vegetarian diets and infant nutrition. Pediatrics. 1982 Oct. 70(44). P. 582-6.

(19)   Wintrobe, et al, <u>Textbook of Internal Medicine</u>, 396-408, McGraw-Hill, New York, NY., 1984.

(20)   Ellis, Frey R., and V.M.E. Montegriffo, "The Health of Vegans, Plant Foods and Human Nutrition." Vol. 2, P. 93-103, 1971. Pergamon Press, Northern Ireland.

(21)   Sanders, T.A.B. (1977) "The Composition of Red Cell Lipid and Adipose Tissue in Vegans, Vegetarians, and Omnivores." Ph.D. Thesis: University of London.

(22)   Sanders, T.A.B. (1982): "An anthropometric and dietary assessment of the nutritional status of vegan preschool children." Journal of Human Nutrition, 35, 349-357.

(23)   Ellis, F.R., et al, "Veganism, Clinical Findings, and Investigations," The American Journal of Clinical Nutrition 23(3): 249, March 1970.

(23a)   Carter, J.P., et al, "Preeclampsia and reproductive performance in a community of vegans." Southern Medical Journal 1987 Jun. 80(6). P. 692-7.

(24)   Journal of the National Cancer Institute, Vo. 51, No. 6, Dec. 1973; and Foreign Agricultural Circular - Livestock and Meat, U.S.D.A., Washington, D.C. 1976.

(25)   Robbins, John, <u>Diet for a New America</u>, Stillpoint Publishers, Walpole, NH, P. 158-167., 1987.

(26)   Lindahl, O., et al, "Vegan regimen with reduced medication in the treatment of bronchial asthma." Journal of Asthma, 1985. 22(1). P. 45-55.

(27)   a. Lucas, P., "Dietary Fat Agravates Active Rheumatoid Arthritis," Clinical Research, 29:754A, 1981.
        b. Parke, A., "Rheumatoid Arthritis and Food..." British Medical Journal, 282:2027, 1981.

(28)   Ellis, F. and Sanders, T., "Angina and Vegan Diet," American Heart Journal, June, 1977, 93:803.

(29)   a. Lithell, H., et al, "A fasting and vegetarian diet treatment trial on chronic inflammatory disorders." Acta-Derm-Venereol (Stockh). 1983. 63(5). P. 397-403.
        b. Beighton, "Rheumatoid Arthritis in a Rural South African Negro Population," Annals of Rheumatic Diseases, 34:136, 1975.

(30)   Reid, J.T., "Comparative Efficiency of Animals in the Conversion of Feedstuffs to Human Foods," Confinement, April 1976, P. 23.

(31)   Roller, W.L., et al, "Energy Costs of Intensive Livestock Production," American Society of Agricultural Engineers, June 1975, St. Joseph, Michigan, paper no. 75-4042, table 7, P. 14, cited in Singer and Mason, Animal Factories, as per note 54.

(32)   a.   Lagrone, William, "The Great Plains" - Report: Nebraska's Water Wealth is Deceptive, Omaha World-Herald, May 28, 1981.

        b.   Harris, Joe, resource economist part of four-year government-sponsored study, "The Six State High Plains Ogallala Aquifer Agricultural Regional Resource Study.", 1987.

(33)   Newsweek, November 8, 1971, P. 85.

(34)   Loehr, Raymond, "Pollution Implications of Animal Wastes - A Forward Oriented Review," Water Pollution Control Research Series, Washington, D.C.: Office of Research and Monitoring, U.S.E.P.A., 1968, P. 26, table 7.

(35)   Reid, J.T., op cit. P. 23.

(36)   a.   Bralove, Mary, "The Food Crisis: the Shortages May Pit the 'Have Nots' Against the 'Haves," Wall Street Journal, October 33, 1974, P. 20.

        b.   Rensberger, Boyce, "World Food Crisis: Basic Ways of Life Face Upheaval from Chronic Shortages," N Y Times, November 5, 1974, P. 14.

(37)   Erlich, Paul and Anne, Population, Resources, Environment, W.H. Freeman, 1972, P. 75-76.

(38)   Parsons, James, "Forest to Pasture: Development or Destruction?" Revista de Biologia Tropical, Vol. 24, Supplement 1, 1976.

(39)   a.   DeWalt, Billie, "The Cattle Are Eating the Forest," Bulletin of the Atomic Scientists.

        b.   The World Conservation Strategy: "The World Conservation Strategy in Brief," World Wildlife Fund, 1980.

(40)   Carter, Vernon Gill, and Dale, Tom, Topsoil and Civilization, Rev. ed., Norman, Univ. of Oklahoma Press, 1974.

(41)   Hur, Robin, "Six Inches from Starvation: How and Why America's Topsoil is Disappearing," Vegetarian Times, March, 1985, P. 45-47.

(42)   Hur, Robin, and Fields, Dr. David, "Are High-Fat Diets Killing Our Forests?" Vegetarian Times, Feb. 1984.

(43)   Hur, Robin and Fields, David, "How Meat Robs America of its Energy," Vegetarian Times, April, 1985.

(44)   Time Magazine, March 26, 1984.

(44a) Statistics from Rand McNally World Almanac, 1987, Military Budget, Page 74.

(45)   Statistics from U. S. Department of Agriculture, Washington, D.C.

(46)   a.   "Chloramphenicol Use by Cattlement Said to be Dangerous," Vegetarian Times, P. 6.

        b.   Schell, Orville, Modern Meat, Random House, New York, NY, P. 278-297.

(47)   a.   Pesticides in Meat - Ibid, P. 150-160.

b. Radioactivity in Beef - Nutrition Week, Vol. XVII, No. 26, June 25, 1987, Community Nutrition Institute, Washington, D.C., P. 2.

(48) a. Keys, A., "Serum Cholesterol Response to Changes in Dietary Lipids," American Journal of Clinical Nutrition, 19:175, 1966.

     b. Sacks, F., op. cit., 292:1148, 1975.

(49) a. Hirayama, T., "Epidemiology of Breast Cancer with Special Reference to the Role of Diet," Preventive Medicine, 7:173, 1978.

     b. Hill, P., "Diet, Life-Style, and Menstrual Activity," American Journal of Clinical Nutrition, 33:1192, 1980 Staszewski, J., "Age at Menarche and Breast Cancer," Journal of the National Cancer Institute, 47:935, 1971.

(50) a. Reddy, B.S., et al, "Nutrition and its Relationship To Cancer," Advances in Cancer Research, 32:237, 1980.

     b. Hill, P., "Environmental Factors of Breast and Prostatic Cancer," Cancer Research, 41:3817, 1981.

(51) Carroll, K., "Experimental Evidence of Dietary Factors and Hormone-Dependent Cancers," Cancer Research, 35:3374, 1975.

(52) Phillips, R., "Role of Lifestyle and Dietary Habits in Risk of Cancer..." Cancer Research, 35:3513, 1975.

(53) Singh, I., "Low-Fat Diet and Therapeutic Doses of Insulin in Diabetes Mellitus," Lancet, 263:422, 1955.

(54) Brenner, op cit 307:652, 1982.

(55) a. Johnson, N., et al, "Effect of Level of Protein Intake in Urinary and Fecal Calcium and Calcium Retention..." Journal of Nutrition, 100:1425, 1970.

     b. Altchuler, S., "Dietary Protein and Calcium Loss: A Review," Nutritional Research, 2:193, 1982.

     c. Hegsted, M., "Urinary Calcium and Calcium Balance in Young Men as Affected by Level of Protein and Phosphorus Intake," Journal of Nutrition, 111:553, 1981.

(56) Op. cit. Ref. 24.

(57) a. Flynn, M., "Serum Lipids in Humans Fed Diets Containing Beef or Fish and Poultry. American Journal of Clinical Nutrition, 34:2734, 1981.

     b. Flynn, M. "Dietary 'meats' and serum lipids." American Journal of Clinical Nutrition, 35:935, 1982.

(58) Ellis, F., et al, "Incidence of Osteopororis in Vegetarians and Omnivores," American Journal of Clinical Nutrition, 25:555, 1972.

(59) a. Fara, G. "Epidemic of Breast Enlargment in an Italina School." Lancet, 2:295, 1979.

     b. Saenz de Rodriguez, C., "Environmental Hormone Contamination in Puerto Rico." New England Journal of Medicine 310:1741, 1984.

(60) "Salmonellae in Slaughter Cattle," Journal of the American Veterinary Medical Association, 160(6):884, 1972.

(61) "Salmonella Contamination in a Commercial Poultry Processing Operation," Poultry Science, 53:814-21, 1974.

(62) Thrash, M.D., Agatha, The Animal Connection, Yucchi Pines Institute, Seale, AL, P. 51.

(63) a. "What Causes Cancer on the Farm?" Medical World News, January 14, 1972, P. 39.

b.   "Intestinal Cancer May Be Increased by Meat Ammonia." Medical Tribune, September 20, 1972.

(64)   "Cancer: From Fowl to Woman?" Time, 83:79, April 3, 1964.

(65)   a.   "Presence of a Carcinogenic Substance in Hens' Eggs." Proceedings of the Society for Experimental Biology and Medicine, 96:332-335, 1957.

b.   Report of the Regional Poultry Research Laboratory. E. Lansing, MI 1949.

(66)   a.   Roberts, S., "Does Egg Feeding (i.e., Dietary Cholesterol) Affect Plasma Cholesterol Levels in Humans? The Results of a Double Blind Study," American Journal of Clinical Nutrition, 34:2092, 1981.

b.   Porter, M., "Effect of Dietary Egg on Serum Cholesterol and Triglyceride of Human Males," American Journal of Clinical Nutrition, 30:490, 1977.

(67)   Op. cit. Ref. 55 & 58.

(68)   Nutrition Week: Community Nutrition Institute, "Salmonella Contamination Linked to Raw Eggs - CDC Atlanta Reports," Vol. XVIII, No. 17, April 28, 1988, Washington, D.C.

(69)   Martin, D.B., et al., "Organochlorine pesticides and polychlorinated biphenyls in sediment and fish from Wetlands in the north central United States." Journal of the Association of Analytical Chemistry, 1985 July-Aug. 68(4). P. 712-7.

(70)   Rainio, K., et al, "Polycyclic aromatic hydrocarbons in mussel and fish from the Finnish Archipelago Sea." Bulletin of Environmental Contamination and Toxicology. 1986 Sept. 37(3). P. 337-43.

(71)   Linsalata, P., et al, "Comparative pathway analysis of radiocesium in the Hudson River Estuary: environmental measurements and regulatory dose assessment models."

(72)   Newsweek, Nov. 16, 1984, P. 48.

(73)   Eisenberg, M., et al., "Organochlorine residues in finfish from Maryland waters 1976-1980." Journal of Environmental Science and Health. 1985 Dec. 20(6). P. 729-42.

(74)   Aly, O.A., et al, "Organochlorine residues in fish from the River Nile, Egypt." Bulletin of Environmental Contamination and Toxicology, 1984 Aug. 33(2). P. 246-52.

(75)   Winger, P.V., "Residues of organochlorine insecticides, polychlorinated biphenyls, and heavy metals in biota from Apalachicola River, Florida, 1978." Journal of the Association of Analytical Chemistry.

(76)   el-Dib, M.A., et al, "Organochlorine insecticides and PCB's in water, sediment, and fish from the Mediterranean Sea." Bulletin of Environmental Contamination and Toxicology. 1985 Feb. 34(2). P. 216-27.

(77)   Falandysz, J., et al, "Total mercury content of the muscles of various species of fish from the Southern Baltic Sea 1982-1983." Rocz-Panstw-Kakl-Hig. 1985. 36(2). P. 119-24.

(78)   "Field and laboratory tests on acute toxicity of cadmium to freshwater crayfish." Bulletin of Environmental Contamination and Toxicology. 1986 Sept. 37(3). P. 355-61.

(79)   Report of "Public Voice for Food and Health Policy" and National Marine Fisheries Service, 1986.

(80)   a.   Airey, D. "Total mercury concentration in human hair from thirteen countries in relation to fish consumption and location." Science of the Total Environment. 1983 Nov. 31(2). P. 157-80.

b.   Takeuchi, T., "Pathology of Minamata disease. With special reference to its pathogenesis." Acta-Pathol-Jpn. 1982. 32 Suppl. 1. P. 73-99. (Review).

(81)   Valciukas, J.A., et al, "Neurobehavioral assessment of Mohawk Indians for subclinical indications of methyl mercury neurotoxicity." Archives of Enviromental Health, 1986 Jul-Aug. 41(4), P. 269-72.

(82)   McKeown, et al, "Methyl mercury exposure in northern Quebec. Neurologic findings in adults." American Journal of Epidemiology. 1983 Oct. 118(4). P. 461-9.

(83)   a. Mykkanen, H., et al, "Dietary intakes of mercury, lead, cadmium and arsenic by Finnish children." Human Nutr. Appl. 1986 Feb. 40(1). P. 32-9.

         b. Boiteau, H.L., et al, "Levels of lead, cadmium and mercury in the hair of inhabitants of the Nantes and Grenoble areas." Toxicol-Eur-Res. 1984 Nov. 5(6). P. 281-91.

(84)   Lommel, A., et al, "Organochlorines and mercury in blood of a fish-eating population at the River Elbe in Schleswig- Holstein, FRG." Arch-Toxicol Suppl. 1985. P. 264-8.

(85)   Swanson, S.M., "Food-chain transfer of U-series radionuclides in a northern Saskatchewan aquatic system." Health Physics. 1985 Nov. 49(5). P. 747-70.

(86)   Czarnezki, J.M., "Accumulation of lead in fish from Missouri streams inpacted by lead mining." Bulletin of Environmental Contamination and Toxicology. 1985 May 34(5). P. 736-45.

(87)   Noren, K., "Levels of organochlorine contaminants in human milk in relation to the dietary habits of the mothers." Acta- Paediatr-Scand. 1983 Nov. 72(6). P. 811-6.

(88)   McDougall's Medicine, John A. McDougall, M.D., New Century Press, P. 254-275, 1986.

(89)   Allen, Lindsay H., Ph.D., et al, "Protein-induced hypercalciuria: a longer term study." The American Journal of Clinical Nutrition 32. April 1979, P. 741-749.

(90)   Marsh, Alice G., et al, "Cortical bone density of adult lacto-ovo-vegetarian and omnivorous women." Journal of the American Dietetic Association. Vol. 76, Feb.1980, P. 148-151.

(91)   Mazess, R., "Bone mineral content of northern Alaskan Eskimos." American Journal of Clinical Nutrition, 27 (1974); 916.

(92)   Vegetarian Sourcebook, Keith Akers. Vegetarian Press. P. 21-50, 1984.

(93)   McDougall, M.D., John, "Fish and Fish Oil are 'Second Line' Therapies." The McDougall Newsletter. Nov.-Dec. 1986.

(94)   Callaway, C. Wayne, "What about fish oil's risks?" Letter to the Washington Post "Health" section, October 14, 1986.

(95)   Carroll, K.K., et al, "Dietary fat and mammary carcinogenesis." Nutrition and Cancer. 1984. 6(4). P. 254-9.

(96)   a. Heaton, K., "Gallstones and Cholecystitis," in Refined Carbohydrate Foods and Diseases, as per note 44.

         b. Sarles, H., "Diet and Cholesterol Gallstones," Digestion, 17:121, 1978.

(97)   Erasmus, Udo, Fats & Oils, Alive Books, Vancouver, B.C., P. 115-135, 1986.

(98)   Sussman, Vic, The Vegetarian Alternative, Rodale Press, Emmaus, PA, 1978, P. 55.

(99)   Hartroft, W., "The Incidence of Coronary Heart Disease in Patients Treated with the Sippy Diet," American Journal of Clinical Nutrition, 15:205, 1964.

(100) a. "When a Child Has Repeated Colds Think of Milk Allergy," Consultant, January, 1968, P. 41.

b. "Milk Has Something for Everybody?" Journal of the American Medical Association 232(5) 539, May 5, 1975.

c. "Recurrent Abdominal Pain in Children: Lactose and Sucrose Intolerance, A Prospective Study." Pediatrics 64:43-45, July, 1979.

(101) Op. cit. Ref. 24.

(102) a. "Unrecognized Disorders Frequently Occurring Among Infants and Children from the Ill Effects of Milk." Southern Medical Journal 31:1016, September, 1938.

b. "Add Milk to Your GI Suspect List." Patient Care, February 15, 1976, P. 116-126.

(103) a. Heaney, R., "Calcium Nutrition and Bone Health in the Elderly," American Journal of Clinical Nutrition, 36:986, 1982.

b. Paterson, C. "Calcium Requirements in Man: A Critical Review," Postgrad Medical Journal, 54:244, 1978.

(104) Recker, R., "The Effect of Milk Supplements on Calcium Metabolism, Bone Metabolism and Calcium Balance," American Journal of Clinical Nutrition, 41:254, 1985.

(105) Wachman, Amnon, et al, "Diet and Osteoporosis," Lancet, May 4, 1968, P. 958.

(106) Nilas, L., "Calcium Supplementation and Postmenopausal Bone Loss," British Medical Journal, 289:1103, 1984.

(107) a. Walker, A., "Osteoporosis and Calcium Deficiency," American Journal of Clinical Nutrition, 16:327, 1965.

b. Smith, R., "Epidemiologic Studies of Osteoporosis in Women of Puerto Rico and Southeastern Michigan..." Clinical Orthopedics 45:32, 1966.

(108) a. "More Clout for Human Cancer Virus." Science News 103:121, February 24, 1973.

b. Thrash, op. cit., P. 41-50.

(109) "Virus-like Particles in Cow's Milk from a Herd with a High Incidence of Lymphosarcoma." Journal of the National Cancer Institute 33:2055-1064, 1964.

(110) "A Multiple Share of Myeloma." Medical World News, May 16, 1969, P. 23.

(111) Op. cit. Ref. 6.

(112) a. Phillips, R., "Coronary Heart Disease Mortality Among Seventh Day Adventists with Differing Dietary Habits," Abstract American Public Health Association Meeting, Chicago, Nov. 16-20, 1975.

b. Op. cit. Thorogood, M.

(113) Op. cit., Moore, M.D., R., P. 20-48.

(114) a. Markakis, P., "The Nutritive Quality of Potato Protein," in Protein Nutritional Quality of Foods and Feeds, pt. 2, ed. M. Friedman, New York: M. Dekker, 1975.

b. Kofranyi, E., et al, "The Minimum Protein Requirement of Humans..." cited in Akers, K., A Vegetarian Sourcebook, G.P. Putnam's Sons, New York, 1983, P. 205.

(115)   Ibid.

(116)   Op. cit. Ref. 9.

(117)   Op. cit. Akers, K., P. 25-30

(118)   Ibid 30-32.

(119)   a.   For corn: C. Kies, E. Williams, and H.M. Fox, "Determination of First Limiting Nitrogenous Factor in Corn
             Protein for Nitrogen Retention in Human Adults," The Journal of Nutrition 86:350, August 1965.

        b.   For wheat: S.B. Vaghefi, et al, "Lysine Supplementation of Wheat Proteins," The American Journal of Clinical
             Nutrition 27:1231, 1974.

        c.   C.J. Lee, et al, "Nitrogen Retention of Young Men Fed Rice With or Without Supplementary Chicken," The
             American Journal of Clinical Nutrition 24:318, 1971.

        d.   P. Markakis, "The Nutritive Quality of Potato Protein," in Protein Nutritional Quality of Foods and Feeds,
             pt. 2, ed. M. Friedman (New York: M. Dekker, 1975).

(120)   Ballentine, M.D., Rudolph, <u>Transition to Vegetarianism</u>, The Himalayan International Institute, Honesdale, PA.,
        P. 269, nt.5.

(121)   Op. cit. Moore, M.D., P. 56-112.

(122)   Op. cit. Ref. 103.

(123)   Op. cit. Allen, L., Ref. 8b.

(124)   Roberts, H. "Potential toxity due to dolomite and bonemeal." Southern Medical Journal 76:556, 1983.

(125)   White, P.I., ed., et al, "Let's Talk About Food" (Acton, MA: Publishing Sciences Group, 1974), P. 211.

(126)   Op. cit. Akers, K., P. 34-38.

(127)   Frey R. Ellis, M.D., et al. "Veganism, Clinical Findings and Investigations." American Journal of Clinical
        Nutrition. Volume 23, #3, March, 1970, P. 249-255.

(128)   Crane, M.D., Milton G., et al. "Vitamin B-12 Studies on Vegans," Weimar Institute, Weimar, CA., 1986.

(129)   Bruce, Gene, "The Myth of Vegetarian B-12," East West Journal, May, 1988, P. 44-55.

(130)   Eisman, George, Journal of North American Vegetarian Society, Volume 12, No. 4, 1985.

(131)   New England Journal of Medicine, March 26, 1981, P. 792.

(132)   a.   Acheson, K., "Carbohydrate Metabolism and De Novo Lipogenesis in Human Obesity," American Journal of
             Clinical Nutrition 45:78, 1987.

        b.   Acheson, K., "Carbohydrate and Liquid Balance," Metabolism, 31:1234, 1982.

(133)   Levin, N., et al. "Energy Intake and Body Weight in Ovo- Lacto Vegetarians." Journal of Clinical
        Gastroenterology. 1986 Aug. 8(4). P. 451-3.

(134) Baker, M.D., Sidney M., Gesell Institute of Human Development Update, Volume 3, No. 2, 1984.

(135) Op. cit. Erasmus, U., P. 107-115.

(136) a. Anderson, J., "High Carbohydrate, High-Fiber Diets for Insulin-Treated Men With Diabetes Mellitus," American Journal of Clinical Nutrition, 32:2312, 1979.

b. Anderson, J., "Hypolipidemic Effects of High- Carbohydrate, High-Fiber Diets," Metabolism, 29:551, 1980.

(137) Kempe, M.D., C. Henry, et al, "Current Pediatric Diagnosis and Treatment," 7th Edition, Lang Medical Publications, 1982, P. 772.

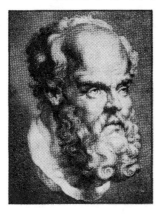

Socrates c470-399

"The highest realms of thought are impossible to reach without first attaining an understanding of compassion."

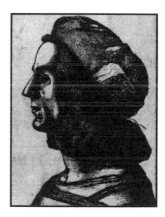

Leonardo da Vinci 1452-1519

"I have from an early age abjured the use of meat, and the time will come when men such as I will look upon the murder of animals as they now look upon the murder of men."

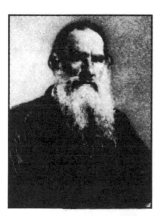

Count Leo Tolstoy 1828-1910

"Vegetarianism serves as the criterion by which we know that the pursuit of moral perfection on the part of humanity is genuine and sincere."

"It often happens that the universal belief of one age, a belief from which no one was free or could be free without an extraordinary effort of genius or courage, becomes to a subsequent age, so palpable an absurdity that the only difficulty is, to imagine how such an idea could ever have appeared credible."

John Stuart Mill
1806-1873

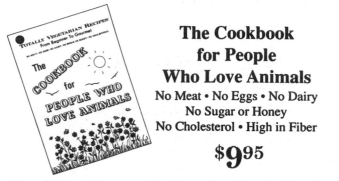
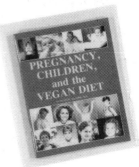
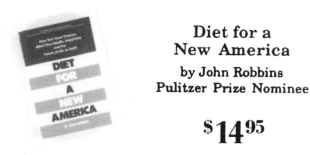
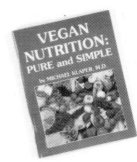
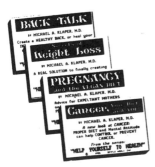